Dementia Handbook

D0278927

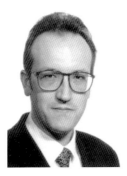

Richard Harvey is an Alzheimer's Disease Society Research Fellow in the Dementia Research Group at the Institute of Neurology, London

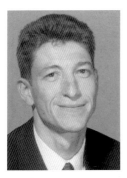

Nick Fox is an MRC Clinician Scientist Fellow and member of the Dementia Research Group at the Institute of Neurology, London

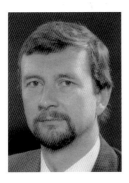

Martin Rossor is Professor of Neurology and Director of the Dementia Research Group at the Institute of Neurology and Imperial College, and Consultant Neurologist at the National Hospital for Neurology and Neurosurgery and St Mary's Hospitals, London

Dementia Handbook

Richard J Harvey MD, MRCPsych

Nick C Fox MA, MRCP

Martin N Rossor MA, MD, FRCP

Dementia Research Group
Institute of Neurology and Division of Neurosciences
Imperial College School of Medicine
The National Hospital for Neurology and Neurosurgery
London WC1N 3BG
UK

Presented with the compliments of
Janssen-Cilag Ltd and Organon

MARTIN DUNITZ

© Martin Dunitz 1999

First published in the United Kingdom in 1999 by

Martin Dunitz Ltd
The Livery House
7–9 Pratt Street
London NW1 0AE

A CIP record for this book is available from the British Library.

ISBN 1-85317-842-X

Composition by Scribe Design, Gillingham, Kent, UK
Printed and bound in Italy.

Contents

Acknowledgements

Richard Harvey is supported by an Alzheimer's Disease Society Research Fellowship. Nick Fox is supported by an MRC Clinician Scientist Fellowship. We wish to extend our gratitude to Dr Angus Kennedy for permission to reproduce the PET images, to Dr Kim Jobst for permission to reproduce temporal lobe CT images, and to Professor Elizabeth Warrington for advice on neuropsychology and permission to reproduce pictures from the Queen Square Screening Tests.

We are grateful for the ongoing support and encouragement of the Dementia Research Group and CANDID in producing this book, in particular Kate Homan, Suzanne Tom, Ron Isaacs, Suzie Barker, Penelope Roques, Jill Walton, Clare Morris, Sandra Beech, Elaine Duncan, Miriam Hall, Lisa Cipolotti, Pam Coward, John Janssen, Rebecca Cordery, John Walters, Rhian Jenkins, Rachael Scahill, Katy Judd and Bill Crum.

Introduction

The dementias pose a major and growing clinical and public health challenge as we enter the twenty-first century. Estimates suggest that as many as one in two of the population who live to the age of 85 years are likely to develop dementia. Although currently a problem mainly affecting the developed world, improvements in public health, and increasing longevity in parts of the developing world mean that, globally, the numbers of dementia sufferers are growing faster than at any time in history.

This pocketbook is aimed directly at the clinician faced with the task of investigating a patient with suspected dementia. Consideration of the full differential diagnosis of dementia can be a complex process – there are no simple diagnostic tests; accurate diagnosis requires experience, clinical skills, the ability to integrate results from a range of tests and the judicious application of clinical diagnostic criteria.

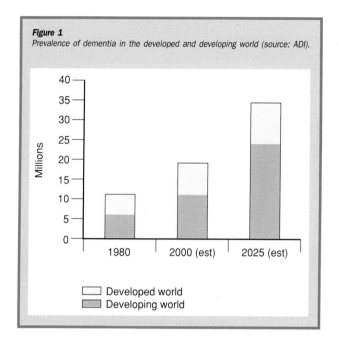

Figure 1
Prevalence of dementia in the developed and developing world (source: ADI).

With the emergence of the first licensed treatments for Alzheimer's disease (AD) the importance of making a specific clinical diagnosis has been underlined for all clinicians investigating patients with dementia. Treatable causes of 'dementia' are no longer confined to the rarities of normal pressure hydrocephalus or frontal meningioma. A simple label of 'dementia' is inadequate; patients with AD can be considered for cholinesterase inhibitor therapy, and the course of vascular dementia may be modified by active intervention aimed at underlying risk factors. A diagnosis of dementia with Lewy bodies may prevent a life-threatening reaction being inadvertently triggered by the use of neuroleptic treatment. Moreover, effective and specific support can only be delivered to patients and caregivers if a name has been put to their disease.

This book is based upon the clinical experience of a psychiatrist and two neurologists, reflecting the multidisciplinary nature of dementia care. It is aimed at consultants, specialist registrars and senior house officers in psychiatry, neurology and elderly medicine, as well as general practitioners with an interest in dementia. It is also hoped that nurses, psychologists, social workers and others involved in the care of people with dementia may find this book a useful source of information on the process of diagnosis, the causes of dementia and the state of the art in management.

We have divided the text into three sections. The first section describes the tools the clinician will need to make the diagnosis; this covers everything from history taking through routine investigations and neuroimaging, to highly specialist tests and investigations that are only likely to be available at regional or national centres. The intention is to present the full battery of tests that are available, together with indications for their application and interpretation of the results derived.

The second section concerns the diagnosis. This systematically covers the major degenerative dementias and some of the unusual dementias that are encountered in clinical practice. We have attempted to summarise briefly the epidemiology for each disease to give some idea of the likely frequency with which it will be found in clinical practice. This is followed by a description of the more common clinical presentations of the disease, appropriate investigations that can support the diagnosis and a summary of the clinical diagnostic criteria.

The final section of the book covers management and includes sections on supporting the patient's caregiver and family, the management of behavioural problems and treatment of specific diseases.

The Tools

Summary

History

Clinical examination
    Psychiatric assessment

Neuropsychological assessment
    Bedside cognitive testing
    Formal neuropsychological assessment

Blood tests
    FBC, ESR, U7E, LFT, Ca⁺, PO₄, thyroid function,
    syphilis serology, vitamin B₁₂, *autoantibodies, C-reactive
    protein, white cell enzymes, heavy metal screen, copper
    studies, HIV, urinary drug screen, tumour markers*

ECG

Chest X-ray

Neuroimaging
    Structural (CT, MRI);
    Functional
    MRA and Doppler ultrasound

EEG

EMG and nerve-conduction studies

Echocardiogram

Examination of the cerebrospinal fluid

Diagnostic genetic testing

Biopsy
   Muscle biopsy
   Tonsillar biopsy
   Cerebral biopsy

Items in bold should be carried out in every case of dementia

History

Careful, methodical and detailed history taking remains the most important part of making the diagnosis in a patient with suspected dementia. Taking the history from the patient alone will usually be unreliable and so it is essential to obtain an independent history from the caregiver, close relative or someone who knows the patient well. Discrepancies in the accounts obtained help to assess the presence and extent of anosognosia (lack of awareness by the patient of their symptoms), an important diagnostic and management feature. The history should include educational and employment background, past medical history, past psychiatric history and a current and past drug history.

A family history is essential, but is potentially distressing to the patient and spouse, and often best left until later in the interview. The family history *must be detailed*; to accept a negative answer to the question, 'Is there a family history of memory impairment?', may overlook an early unrelated death in the family in which there is an autosomal dominant dementia.

The cognitive history needs to explore the different cognitive domains, e.g. forgetting items, getting lost, not recognising familiar faces, word-finding difficulties and other changes in language, dressing problems, calculation etc. Changes in the family role, e.g. shopping and housework taken on by the husband or finances by the wife, is an important early clue, particularly as in the elderly age group such labour divisions based upon gender are usual. Changes in personality, which may include eating behaviour, sexual activity, clothing choice and the social graces are important, but delicate, issues. These will usually need to be enquired of the informant in the absence of the patient. Useful opportunities arise whilst the patient is undressing in the examination room or while they are undergoing some other investigation. For example, characteristic behavioural features of the semantic dementias include changes in sexual behaviour (both increased and decreased libido), overdressing, change in food preference and quantity, ritual-istic behaviours and excessive religious interest ('hypereligiosity').

The chronological progression of symptoms should be carefully documented from the very earliest clue that the patient was becoming cognitively impaired, through major functional watersheds such as the patient or caregiver having to give up work, to the appearance of behavioural problems. It is important to get a clear picture of the initial symptoms. Were memory difficulties the very first changes noticed? Was the course gradual and insidiously progressive? Have there been step-wise deteriorations? Are there significant day-to-day fluctuations? It can be helpful to understand the patient's current functional abilities and disabilities by encouraging the informant to describe the patient's typical daily activities.

Finally, it is critically important to enquire and record in the medical notes whether the patient drives and whether they have had any accidents. A useful question is whether the informant feels safe in the passenger seat with the patient driving. The issue of driving is covered in more detail in Section 3.

Clinical examination

General physical examination is important with a specific focus on cardiac assessment. Any patient with dementia who has not been undressed has not been examined properly.

The examination of the patient with possible cognitive decline may be conveniently divided into four parts:

- The mental state
- Cognition
- Neurological examination
- General examination.

In practice, these assessments overlap, and findings in one are should direct later aspects of the examination. For example, prominent visual hallucinations should prompt careful examination for extrapyramidal signs (LBD) while slow 'subcortical' responses to cognitive testing would focus attention on peripheral signs and causes of cerebrovascular disease.

A careful general neurological examination is important, even if frequently found to be normal. The examination begins with the first contact with the patient, where clues to the diagnosis can often be gained by watching the patient come into the consulting room. The following schema is not exhaustive but is aimed at points that require particular attention.

Gait

Examination of the patient's gait is very helpful. Difficulty in getting up out of a chair may suggest dypraxia or extrapyramidal problems. A shuffling gait with small steps, with difficulty in starting or stopping, may be due to extrapyramidal disease. However, if the problems with gait are combined with relatively little in the way of extrapyramidal features in the arms, face and speech then this 'lower body Parkinsonism' is a pointer to small vessel cerebrovasacular disease. *Marche à petit pas* is the term given to a short-stepped gait with good arm swing and upright (not Parkinsonian) posture and, while this may be produced by frontal lobe tumours or degeneration, it is also seen in small vessel vascular dementia. An unsteady shuffling gait, with difficulty in initiation and turning, may be part of the triad of gait disturbance, incontinence and dementia seen in hydrocephalus A; a wide-based ataxic gait suggests cerebellar involvement (CJD; alcohol-related cerebellar degeneration). If the patient appears disproportionately unsteady (e.g. brought in in a wheelchair), consider progressive supranuclear palsy (PSP) where early falls are common. While the patient is getting up and walking is a good time to observe for abnormal movements – a wandering dystonic arm, indicating corticobasal degeneration, or choreiform movements, suggesting Huntington's disease.

Vision and eye movements

The fundi should be examined, together with the visual fields, looking for field defects or visual disorientation. Visual disorientation may often be suspected from the history; such patients, when asked to touch your hand in the peripheral visual field, may often touch your face or take hold of your tie ('the tie sign').

Eye movements are important and may be difficult to elicit in moderately demented patients; patients are often able to follow your face if unable to follow the hand. Saccadic pursuit movements (i.e. jerky movements on following an object) suggest additional cerebellar dysfunction. A discrepancy between voluntary saccadic movements and pursuit may be seen if the patient is unable to follow instructions. However, improvement of saccadic movements, especially vertical, with preservation of occulocephalic movements (i.e. moving the head whilst gaze is fixed on an object) suggests a diagnosis of PSP (Steele–Richardson syndrome). A similar picture can be seen in Niemann–Pick disease type C.

Motor function

Facial asymmetry and weakness should be looked for. Assessment of the quality of the patient's speech is most efficiently performed when language skills are tested. A slurring dysarthria is common in PSP, while a pseudo-bulbar palsy may point to motor neurone disease or cerebrovascular disease. Test the jaw jerk and look for evidence of orofacial dyspaxia (a difficulty in tongue protrusion, yawning, blowing or coughing to command, which sometimes results in the patient saying the word 'cough' when attempting to perform the action). Dysphagia should also be enquired about and may be tested by asking the patient to take a small drink of water. The facial

reflexes/pout and jaw jerk should be tested: brisk reflexes suggest cerebrovascular disease.

Care needs to be taken in determining release phenomenon. It is common to misinterpret increased facial reflexes (pout) as a primitive or rooting reflex. Oral puckering in response to a visual stimulus is more reliable, as is utilisation behaviour. Utilisation behaviour is a dramatic demonstration of environmental dependency, e.g. if given a pair of spectacles a patient will put them on, if given another pair these will also be put on, sometimes until 3 or 4 pairs are stacked.

Tone needs to be assessed carefully but, again, this can be difficult. *Gegenhalten* is very common in patients with dementia and does not necessarily reflect extra-pyramidal involvement. Every patient needs to be examined carefully for fasciculation, which is seen most commonly over the deltoids in patients with the MND (motor neurone disease) variant of FTD (frontotemporal dementia).

Table 1 summarises abnormal signs found on physical examination that can be helpful in the different diagnosis of dementia.

Table 1
Abnormal signs found during physical examination that aid in the differential diagnosis of dementia.

Finding on clinical examination	Significance in differential diagnosis of dementia
Hypertension	One of the most significant risk factors for vascular dementia; need further assessment and evaluation of other vascular factors.
Evidence of heart disease (murmurs, signs of cardiac failure)	May suggest a source of emboli in multi-infarct vascular dementia. Needs further investigation with echocardiography.
Carotid bruits	Suggests carotid stenosis, as a source of emboli in vascular dementia.
General malaise, cachexia or lymphadenopathy	Consider a malignancy or HIV.
Hepatosplenomegaly, or other stigmata of liver disease	Seen in a variety of disorders that suggest disease is secondary to a systemic disorder. This may be seen particularly with hepatic encephalopathy, malignant disease and rarities, such as lysosomal storage disorders.
Presence of primitive reflexes (e.g. rooting and grasping reflexes)	Common in severe dementias of all types. Appear early in patients with frontotemporal dementia.
Extensor plantar response (upgoing)	Upper motor neurone signs are not a feature of the degenerative dementias until late in the disease, but are commoner with vascular dementia and should raise suspicion of a structural or metabolic lesion. In the elderly, extensor plantar responses are commonly seen with co-existent spondylitic cervical myelopathy.
Muscle fasciculation – most commonly seen over the deltoid muscle, but may be seen elsewhere	Suggests anterior horn cell disease in the spinal cord. Most commonly seen in motor neurone disease; in a patient with cognitive impairment, suggests the motor neurone variant of frontotemporal dementia. Further investigation with EMG is useful to confirm diagnosis.

Table 1
Continued

Finding on clinical examination	Significance in differential diagnosis of dementia
Eye movements	Eye movements are difficult to test as dementia severity increases. Early presentations with impaired pursuit or nystagmus suggest cerebellar or metabolic (e.g. drug intoxication) disturbance. A supranuclear palsy suggests a diagnosis of progressive supranuclear palsy (PSP).
Myoclonus	Intermittent twitching and jumping movements of the muscles. Seen in CJD and patients with young onset and particularly familial AD. May also be seen in Huntington's disease.
Extrapyramidal features: akinetic-rigidity	Suggests Parkinson's disease (PD), dementia with Lewy bodies (DLB), PSP or corticobasal degeneration. It may also be due to the use of neuroleptic drugs. An asymmetrical pill-rolling tremor suggests PD.
Dyspraxia	Common to many dementias in later stages: in AD it is usually bilateral; in corticobasal degeneration it is unilateral, usually initially involving one arm. Ask patient to copy hand gestures and mime simple actions.
Gegenhalten	Found commonly in dementia. A resistance to passive movement that can be decreased by distraction and is not consistently increased by contralateral movement.
Alien limb phenomenon	The patient will often report that an arm or leg has a 'life of its own' and is almost always asymmetrical; on examination, the limb may move and even grasp objects involuntarily. Best assessed by distracting the patient with some other task and observing the limb. Seen in corticobasal degeneration.
Utilisation behaviour	A dramatic sign associated with frontal lobe disorders.

Psychiatric assessment

All patients with dementia should have at least a basic assessment of their mental state. Psychiatric symptoms are not always spontaneously reported either by the patient or the informant yet they can often provide important clues to the diagnosis. Symptoms, such as depression and psychosis, are major determinants of caregiver burden and are often amenable to treatment once they are recognised.

It is helpful to divide the psychopathology of dementia into six domains, which can form the basis of a systematic enquiry:

- Personality change
- Delusions
- Hallucinations
- Mood and affect disorder
- Neurovegetative change
- Troublesome behaviour.

Personality change

The most common changes in the personality that occur in dementia are disengagement, apathy and disinhibition. Personality changes represent subtle alterations in the way the patient behaves and interacts with other people. In FTD, personality changes can be the earliest symptoms and may pre-date cognitive change by many years. Documenting personality change requires careful history taking from a reliable informant who must have known the patient for many years. Disengagement and apathy are common in AD, vascular dementia (VaD) and dementia with Lewy bodies (DLB), while disinhibition is common in frontotemporal dementia (FTD).

Delusions

Delusions are false beliefs and are a common feature of dementia (Harvey, 1996). The delusional ideas experienced by patients with dementia are rarely as complex or systematised as those of patients with functional psychotic illness, but are usually more simple or concrete false beliefs. The most common delusions experienced by patients with dementia are summarised below.

- Theft
- Persecution and endangerment
- Infidelity of spouse
- One's home is not one's home
- Abandonment
- Capgras' syndrome (*belief that the spouse or other friend or relative has been replaced by an impostor who looks like the spouse/friend/ relative*)
- De Clerambault's syndrome (*false belief that another person, often someone famous or not personally known to the patient, is in love with the patient*)
- Parasitosis (*delusional infestation*)
- Phantom boarder (*the false belief that there are one or more other people living in the house with the patient*)
- Picture sign (*the false belief that the patient's reflection in a mirror is not the patient, but is some other person. Possibly a secondary delusion based upon mis-perception or self-prosopagnosia*).

Hallucinations

Hallucinations can occur in any one of the five sensory modalities, which include, in descending order of frequency of occurrence: visual; auditory; gustatory; olfactory; and tactile hallucinations. Eliciting the presence of hallucinations requires questioning of the patient and caregiver, and particular attention must be paid to the time of day and the setting in which the experiences occur. Hallucinations are a particular features of DLB, and may occur dramatically in the context of rapid eye movement (REM) or non-REM parasomnias, where the patient awakes from a particular phase of sleep and experiences vivid hallucinations.

Mood and affect disorder

Depressed mood and clinical depression are common to all dementias. Differentiating disengagement and apathy from depressive symptoms can be difficult. It is, however, important to identify and treat clinical depression since this can dramatically improve the patient's functional abilities, and both the patient and caregiver's quality of life. The use of a simple depression rating scale, such as the BASDEC (Adshead et al, 1992), Geriatric Depression Scale or Cornell Scale of Depression in Dementia (Alexopoulous et al, 1988) can be a very helpful part of a formalised assessment. Elevation of mood towards hypomania is less common and may be difficult to differentiate from disinhibition in FTD.

In Section 3 we discuss further the management of depression in dementia.

Neurovegetative change

Neurovegetative change covers sleep disorders, eating disorders and changes in sexual behaviour. Sleep disorders include increases or decreases in the amount of sleep, fragmentation of sleep patterns, day–night reversal with nocturnal arousal and nightmares.

Many patients with dementia alter their dietary preferences, yet as these changes can be subtle they are often not reported spontaneously. The most common dietary change is towards a preference for sweet foods, which can be dramatic in FTD. Changes in appetite can lead to both over-eating with weight gain, or under-eating with associated weight loss. Pica type syndromes have also been reported with patients eating non-food items, or unpalatable foodstuff, such as pet foods or raw meat.

Changes in sexual behaviour include increases, decreases and even complete disappearance of libido, changes in preference for the sexual object, such as the development of fetishism and paedophilia. This is inevitably a sensitive area; caregivers, however, are often keen to talk about these types of symptoms, and yet are often unable to raise the subject spontaneously.

Troublesome behaviour

Troublesome behaviour is, to some extent, an umbrella term that encompasses all those more complex behaviours that cannot be fitted into any of the above categories. The most common types of troublesome behaviours are as follows:

- Psychomotor restlessness – pacing, wandering
- Psychomotor retardation
- Stereotypic and repetitive behaviour
- Aggression – verbal and/or physical.

It is inevitably easier to talk to the informant about these symptoms in the absence of the patient. Using a simple ABC (Antecedents, Behaviour, Consequences) behavioural framework to explore symptoms in this area can be particularly worthwhile. We discuss the management of behaviour problems in greater detail in Section 3.

Neuropsychological examination

Neuropsychological examination is the first key investigation of dementia and is used to document the pattern and degree of deficits in the various domains of cognitive function. These domains have a direct relationship to specific brain structures and areas, and can therefore be used to map the pattern and distribution of disease. Neuropsychological assessment falls broadly into two categories – bedside testing, which should be performed routinely by the clinician, and the formal assessment, which is usually carried out by a neuropsychologist.

Bedside cognitive testing

At its most basic, bedside cognitive testing should include an assessment such as the MMSE (Mini Mental State Examination) (Folstein et al, 1975), which grades the patient's cognitive state. While this gives an indication of the degree of cognitive impairment, it provides minimal information about the pattern of deficits – which is the most useful information in differential diagnosis. Longer and more detailed assessments, such as the CAMDEX (Roth et al, 1986) and its associated cognitive test CAMCOG, can provide domain-specific information on cognitive impairment, yet it is not a tool for routine use and probably only has a place in settings such as a memory clinic.

Bedside tests should explore the major cognitive domains in a systematic manner. For example, the Queen Square Screening Test for Cognitive Deficits (Warrington, 1989) is a pocket-sized companion for cognitive testing, which provides a set of comprehensive, structured test materials covering nearly all domains of cognitive function:

- Orientation and alterness
- Language skills
- Literacy skills
- Praxic skills
- Memory
- Perceptual skills.

The test is particular helpful in providing both verbal and visual materials (**see Figure 2**), which are often lacking in other tests, and ensures coverage of both left and right hemisphere function. Unlike the MMSE and CAMCOG there are no normative values since the intention is to provide the clinician with a tool to explore cognition, rather than to replace the quantitative assessment of a neuropsychologist.

The assessment of memory, in particular, should address short- and long-term memory, memory for events (episodic memory), memory for meaning (semantic memory) and procedural memory. For example, episodic memory impairment is a key early feature of AD, while semantic memory impairment may be a feature of FTD.

Formal neuropsychological assessment

The role of the neuropsychologist is to quantify and interpret the pattern and degree of cognitive deficit in the patient with suspected dementia. The specific tests used by psychologists will inevitably vary from centre to centre. However, for the clinician the most important factor is the presentation of the results and, particularly, how this is used to describe the pattern of deficit.

Neuropsychological assessment usually starts with an assessment that estimates pre-morbid intelligence, such

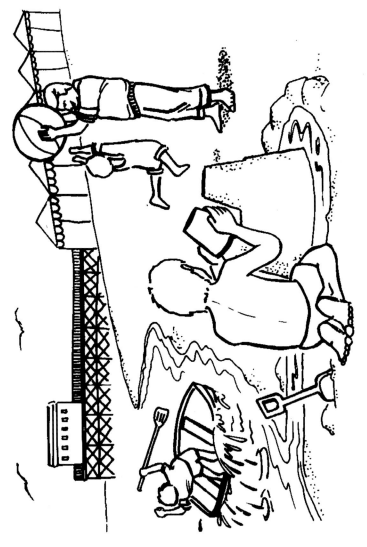

(A)

Figure 2
Pictorial material from The Queen Square Screening Tests for Cognitive Deficits. (A) Picture description: helpful in the general assessment of language; visual perception; naming; and visual memory. Reproduced with permission of Professor EK Warrington (see references for details of how to obtain this test).

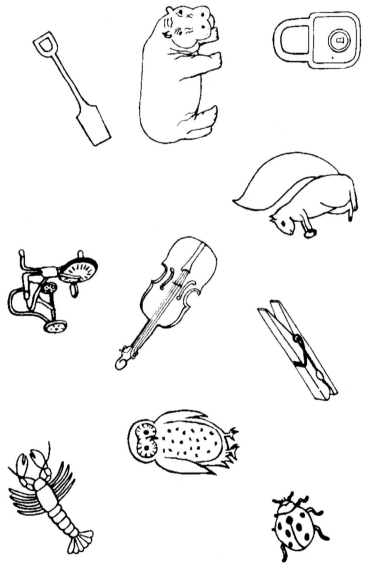

(B)

Figure 2 continued
Pictorial material from The Queen Square Screening Tests for Cognitive Deficits. (B) Objects for language assessment (naming) and visual memory. Reproduced with permission of Professor EK Warrington (see references for details of how to obtain this test).

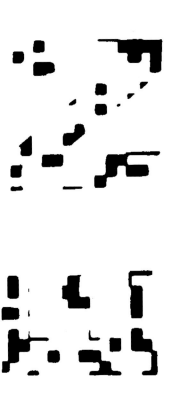

(C)

Figure 2 continued
Pictorial material from The Queen Square Screening Tests for Cognitive Deficits. (C) Fragment letters for assessing visual perception. Reproduced with permission of Professor EK Warrington (see references for details of how to obtain this test).

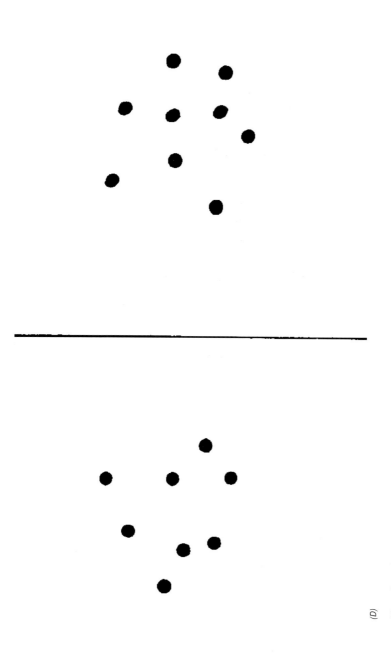

(D)

Figure 2 continued

Pictorial material from The Queen Square Screening Tests for Cognitive Deficits. (D) Dot counting: a useful test for visual disorientation. Reproduced with permission of Professor EK Warrington (see references for details of how to obtain this test).

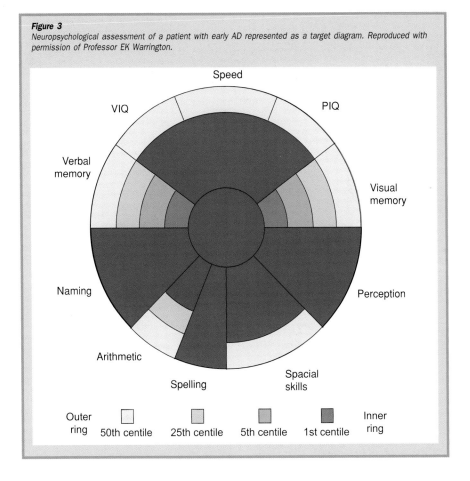

Figure 3
Neuropsychological assessment of a patient with early AD represented as a target diagram. Reproduced with permission of Professor EK Warrington.

as the National Adult Reading Test (NART) (Nelson, 1991), which, when interpreted with information on educational attainment, provides a good indication of optimum function. An estimate of current verbal (dominant hemisphere) and performance (non-dominant hemisphere) IQ is then made using the Wechsler Adult Intelligence Scale (WAIS) (Wechsler, 1981). A discrepancy between the estimated and current IQ suggests a decline in intelligence, supporting the diagnosis of dementia in the absence of other clear causes for this discrepancy.

A range of domain-specific and lateralising tests can then be used to map the pattern of deficits. A basic battery would cover verbal and visual memory, language, visuo-perceptual and visuospatial skills and frontal executive function. In each of these areas, tests should be chosen on the basis of being of graded difficulty and having well-validated age-related normal values, with the exception of frontal executive function tests where these are less satisfactory. By using well-validated graded-difficulty tests, the patient's score can be corrected to a percentile score that indicates their relative level of functioning in comparison to the normal population. For example, a patient's score can be interpreted as being below the 50th, 25th, 5th or 1st percentile. A performance below the 5th percentile is usually taken as

evidence of significant impairment on the test.

Representing the results from each domain as percentile scores provides a simple and easily assimilated method for mapping and displaying the pattern and degree of deficits. The scores can be arranged in the form of a 'target' diagram, as developed by Professor Elizabeth Warrington, with the sectors of the target organised in an approximately anatomical arrangement. **Figure 3** presents the results of a neuropsychological assessment of a patient with AD. In this assessment the patient's speed, performance IQ, verbal IQ and spatial skills are at the 50th percentile, while arithmetic skills are at the 25th percentile, and memory, bilaterally, is below the 1st percentile. Naming, perception and spelling are all still above the 50th percentile. The target diagram clearly displays this pattern, which, for this patient, is known to be associated with AD. We will describe other characteristic patterns of deficit in Section 2.

Blood tests

Clinicians commonly refer to a range of blood tests as being a 'dementia screen', although opinions on which specific tests should be included vary from unit to unit. As with other areas of medicine, a 'screen of tests' is rarely so productive as those directed by the history and examination. **Table 2** sets out the first- and second-line tests that can assist the diagnosis in dementia. Beyond the second line of tests other investigations might be indicated, and often specialist advice will be needed on the interpretation of these results. For each test we have tried to set out the common indications and, wherever possible, some interpretation of an abnormal result in the context of a patient with cognitive impairment. In general, more extensive investigations are needed for younger patients and for those with 'dementia plus' syndromes, i.e. cognitive impairment in the setting of systemic disease or additional neurological symptoms and signs.

Table 2
First- and second-line blood tests that assist in the differential diagnosis of dementia.

Test	Indication	Interpretation in cognitive impairment
Full blood count	All patients	A simple routine test to exclude anaemia, polycythaemia, and other markers of systemic disease that may result in cognitive impairment.
Erythrocyte sedimentation rate (ESR)	All patients	The ESR is a non-specific marker of inflammation. In the absence of a systemic cause for a raised ESR it may suggest central nervous system (CNS) inflammation, such as in a cerebral vasculitis. A raised ESR in a cognitively impaired patient would be an indication for CSF examination and further investigation. A raised ESR in the elderly with cognitive impairment also raises the suspicion of cranial (temporal) arteritis.
Urea and electrocytes, liver function tests, calcium and phosphate	All patients	These simple screening tests should always be performed as part of the process of excluding systemic causes for cognitive inpairment. γ-GT is important as a marker of alcohol abuse. A raised calcium level may suggest metastatic bone disease.
Thyroid function tests	All patients	It is important to exclude hyper- and hypothyroidism as contributory factors to cognitive impairment.

Table 2
Continued

Test	Indication	Interpretation in cognitive impairment
Syphilis serology	All patients	The TPHA (*Treponema Pallidum* Haemagglutination Assay) or FTA (Fluorescent Tremponemal Antibody) tests are highly specific markers of syphillitic infection and remain positive for life, even after treatment. The VDLR (Venereal Disease Research Laboratory) test is a marker of active infection. A positive VDLR with neurological signs would be an indication for CSF syphillis serology and, if positive, urgent treatment or referral to a venereal diseases or microbiology expert.
Serum vitamin B₁₂	All patients	To exclude a deficiency state. Although rarely relevant to cognitive impairment, even mild deficiencies should probably be treated.
Autoantibody screen	Younger patients and those with raised inflammatory markers or anaemia.	The main autoantibodies of importance in the investigation of dementia are anti-nuclear antibody (SLE), anti-thyroid micro-somal antibody (Hashimotos encephalopathy), anti-cardiolipin antibody (anti-phospholipid syndrome and vascular disease), andanti-soluble RNA antibody (scleroderma vasculopathy).
C-reactive protein	Suspicion of an inflammatory process, e.g. raised ESR	C-reactive protein is raised in acute infection and inflammation. It may support evidence of CNS inflammation.

continued overleaf

Table 2
Continued

Test	Indication	Interpretation in cognitive impairment
White cell enzymes	Younger patients, particularly with 'dementia plus' syndromes	Reduced arylsulphatase activity in white cells supports a diagnosis of meta-chromatic leukodystrophy. Although rare, it may present as dementia, with delusions, dystonia, ataxia, nystagmus, seizures and perpheral neuropathy. Hexosaminidase A is reduced in the GM2 gangliosidoses that may present with adult-onset neurological syndromes.
Heavy metal screen	Suspected heavy metal poisoning	If there is an suspicion of heavy metal poisoning, accidental, occupational or deliberate, then a heavy metal screen should be performed.
Copper studies	Suspicion of Wilson's disease	Wilson's disease is associated with accumulation of copper, with degeneration of the liver and brain. The disease can present with a slow, insidious dementia. Other features include hepatosplenomegaly and Kayser–Fleischer rings on slit-lamp examination of the cornea.
HIV	In suspected HIV infection	If there us any suspicion of risk of HIV infection then HIV testing should be carried out with appropriate counselling and consent.
Urinary drug screen	In suspected drug intoxication	
Tumour markers	In suspected paraneoplastic syndromes	Paraneoplastic syndromes, such as limbic encephalitis and Lambert–Eaton syndrome, may present with cognitive impairment.
Genetic testing		See later

Systemic investigations

Electrocardiogram

The majority of patients with dementia, particularly the elderly, should have a routine 12-lead electrocardiogram (ECG) as part of their clinical assessment. The ECG can demonstrate arrhythmias and conduction deficits any of which may be a contributing factor to the cognitive impairment and should be fully investigated.

A 24-hour, or serial 24-hour ECGs are occasionally required in patients with cognitive impairment who are also experiencing blackouts.

Chest X-ray

A routine chest X-ray is an important investigation for the exclusion of systemic pathology, particularly in more elderly patients.

Neuroimaging

Just as neuropsychology can demonstrate the pattern and degree of cognitive deficit, so structural neuroimaging is able to show the pattern and degree of cerebral atrophy, and functional neuroimaging can show patterns of metabolic deficit and changes in neurotransmitter receptors. Structural imaging is important for excluding secondary causes of dementia, e.g. tumours, hydrocephalus, etc.

Structural neuroimaging

Structural neuroimging should be considered for all patients with cognitive impairment. The availability of structural neuroimaging for patients with dementia in many units remains highly restricted; however, for patients of any age, the suspicion of a subdural haemorrhage, cerebral tumour or focal neurological sign would be an absolute indication for imaging.

Beyond the exclusion of major treatable intracranial pathologies, increasing clinical experience and

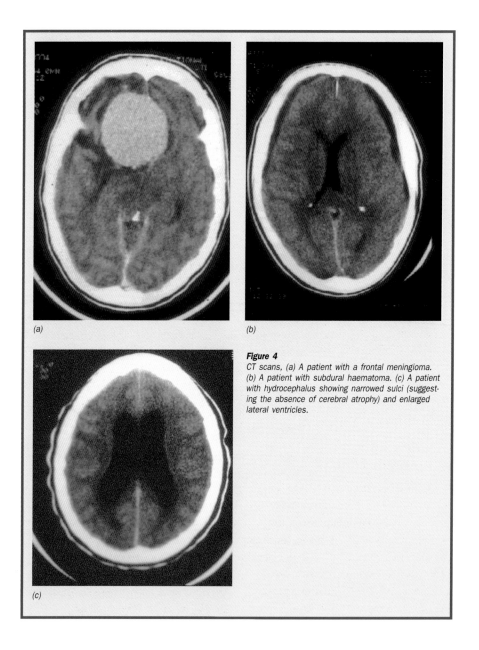

(a)

(b)

(c)

Figure 4
CT scans, (a) A patient with a frontal meningioma.
(b) A patient with subdural haematoma. (c) A patient
with hydrocephalus showing narrowed sulci (suggesting the absence of cerebral atrophy) and enlarged
lateral ventricles.

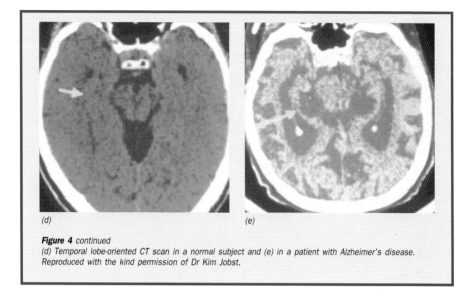

(d)   *(e)*

Figure 4 *continued*
(d) Temporal lobe-oriented CT scan in a normal subject and (e) in a patient with Alzheimer's disease. Reproduced with the kind permission of Dr Kim Jobst.

research suggests that neuroimaging, particularly magnetic resonance imaging (MRI), has a major role to play in the diagnosis of dementia and monitoring of disease progression.

Computed tomography

Computed tomography (CT) scanning is based upon X-ray technology and produces relatively inexpensive, low-resolution images of the brain, usually in the axial plane. CT images do not have such good soft-tissue contrast as MRI, and can also suffer from artefact near the bony structures; they also expose patients to a moderate dose of radiation. CT is the investigation of choice in suspected acute subarachnoid haemorrhage, and is the only neuroimaging technique available to patients with cardiac pacemakers, and intraocular or intracranial metallic foreign bodies. Some patients, who are unable to tolerate MRI scanning due to claustrophobia, may be able to tolerate a CT head scan. **Figure 4** shows example CT scans from patients with a frontal meningioma, subdural haematoma, normal-pressure hydrocephalus, and a temporally orientated CT scan used to assess the size of medial temporal lobe structures.

Magnetic resonance imaging

Magnetic resonance imaging (MRI) is becoming the most important imaging technique for the differential diagnosis of dementia. When compared with CT it has better resolution, better soft-tissue contrast and reveals anatomical features of the brain that are important in the diagnosis of dementia. Examples include visualising medial temporal lobe structures to support a diagnosis of AD, demonstrating focal cortical atrophy to support a diagnosis of FTD, and vascular or ischaemic lesions and infarcts to support a diagnosis of VaD (Fox et al, 1995; Jack, 1998). Formatting the scan as coronal images is particularly helpful in assessing scans from patients with dementia. **Figure 5** shows MR scans from a range of patients demonstrating how the scan findings can support the diagnosis.

Functional neuroimaging

The three functional imaging techniques that have been applied to dementia are PET (Positron Emission Tomography), SPECT (Single Positron Emission Computed Tomography) and fMRI (Functional MRI). PET can be used to evaluate cerebral glucose or oxygen metabolism as markers of brain cell activity or metabolism, using rapidly decaying radiolabelled oxygen or glucose **Figure 6**. SPECT provides an estimate of cerebral perfusion using a radiolabelled tracer. Resolution of both types of scan is low, and can barely resolve an area of brain the size of the hippocampus. PET scans are very costly due to the requirement of the cyclotrom to generate the isotopes, making it almost exclusively a research tool.

Although SPECT is much cheaper it is only semi-quantitative and, moreover, it can only be used as an adjunct to structural imaging and thus its place in clinical practice remains unclear. Functional MRI and MR spectroscopy are alternative methods of assessing cerebral metabolism, although they currently remain research tools with an unclear role in clinical practice.

There is no evidence to support the routine use of functional neuroimaging in the diagnosis of dementia, although Kennedy (1998) has proposed four situations where it may be useful:

1. In very mildly cognitively impaired individuals where a diagnosis is not clear, a characteristic pattern of functional deficit may support a

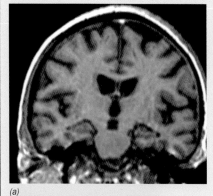

(a)

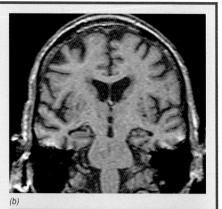

(b)

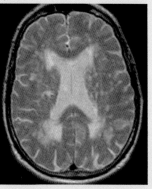

(c)

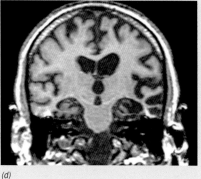

(d)

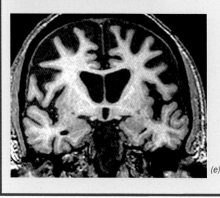

(e)

Figure 5
(a) Coronal MRI in Alzheimer's disease showing global atrophy with ventricular dilatation and tissue loss from the hippocampi. (b) Coronal T1-weighted MRI from a patient with vascular dementia showing atrophy and punctate infarcted areas. (c) Axial T2-weighted MRI from the same patient as in (b) showing high signal intensity white-matter lesions (infarcts). (d) Coronal T1-weighted MRI of a patient with Pick's disease, type FTD, showing the characteristic focal left temporal lobe atrophy. (e) Coronal T1-weighted MRI of a patient with frontal type FTD, showing dramatic focal frontal lobe atrophy.

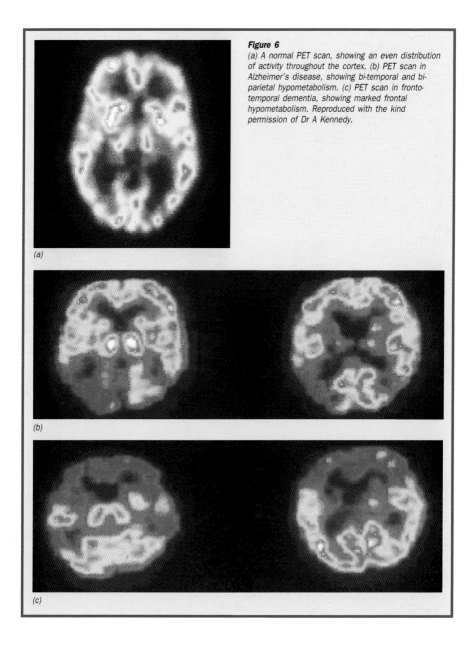

Figure 6
(a) A normal PET scan, showing an even distribution of activity throughout the cortex. (b) PET scan in Alzheimer's disease, showing bi-temporal and bi-parietal hypometabolism. (c) PET scan in fronto-temporal dementia, showing marked frontal hypometabolism. Reproduced with the kind permission of Dr A Kennedy.

(a)

(b)

(c)

specific diagnosis (e.g. a temporoparietal deficit would support a diagnosis of AD).

2. To confirm a clinical diagnosis of AD, particularly early in the disease.

3. To confirm a diagnosis of FTD particularly early in the disease when only behavioural symptoms may be present. A characteristic frontal metabolic deficit would support the diagnosis.

4. In patients with focal neuropsychological deficits but normal structural imaging, a pattern of hypometabolism compatible with the psychological deficits would support the diagnosis of a degenerative process.

Magnetic resonance angiography and doppler ultrasound

Both magnetic resonance angiography (MRA) and doppler ultrasound can be used to image extracranial and large intracranial vessels for stenosis. MR angiography is a very safe technique that uses MRI with virtually no need for contrast angiography in the investigation of suspected vascular causes of cognitive impairment.

Neurophysiology

Electroencephalography

The electroencephalogram (EEG) records the electrical activity of the brain from scalp electrodes over a period of 10–30 minutes. The EEG can be particularly helpful in a number of situations when investigating a patient with dementia. Classically the EEG changes seen in AD and VaD are a generalised slowing represented by reduction or even disappearance of alpha activity with the appearance of theta and delta rhythms. These changes are unfortunately usually seen only once the disease is clearly established, and when the diagnosis is clear.

However, in early disease the EEG can be useful in three ways:

1. Temporal lobe epileptiform spikes have been shown to be the cause of isolated memory deficits in some patients, who respond to therapy with anticonvulsants.

Figure 7
Pseudoperiodic sharp-wave activity on the EEG in sporadic CJD.

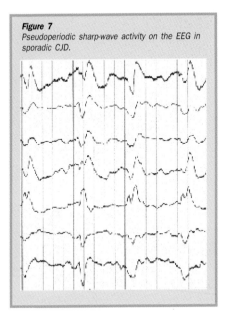

A sleep EEG, particularly when combined with video recording, can be especially helpful in patients with behavioural syndromes, particularly hallucinations, associated with sleep. REM and non-REM parasomnias can be diagnosed and are often amenable to treatment.

Electromyelogram and nerve-conduction studies

An electromyelogram (EMG) is indicated in patients with dementia who have evidence of muscle fasciculation on clinical examination. The EMG can demonstrate denervation and help to confirm a diagnosis of MND type FTD.

2. A normal EEG in the presence of frontal and frontotemporal neuropsychological deficits or frontal behavioural change is supportive of a diagnosis of FTD.

3. In sporadic Creutzfeldt–Jakob disease (CJD) the EEG shows characteristic pseudoperiodic sharp-wave activity (**Figure 7**) which is diagnostic, but present in only 70% of cases. If CJD is suspected but the EEG is negative, the classical changes may show up on serial EEGs.

Nerve conduction studies are indicated when there is evidence of a peripheral neuropathy, e.g. with vitamin B_{12} deficiency or metachromatic leuko-dystrophy.

Echocardiogram

Patients with suspected VaD, particularly if there is evidence of infarcts on neuroimaging, should undergo an echocardiogram to exclude a treatable source of emboli.

Examination of the cerebrospinal fluid

Examination of the cerebrospinal fluid (CSF) remains an important investigation in dementia, particularly in younger patients, and any patient with atypical progressing disease, in whom one might suspect a CNS inflammatory condition. Psychiatrists are unlikely to have the skills and facilities required to carry out routine lumbar punctures (LP); however, it is important to consider whether an LP is indicated and to seek advice and assistance from neurologist or physician colleagues if it is.

Table 3 summarises the important CSF findings and their relevance to patients with cognitive impairment.

Table 3
CSF findings and their relevance to patients with cognitive impairment.

Parameter	Normal finding	Significance of abnormality in dementia
Appearance	Clear and colourless	Blood in the CSF suggests haemorrhage into the subarachnoid space, with xanthochromia (yellow) colour persisting for several weeks after a bleed.
Pressure	5–15 cm H_2O with patient recumbent	Raised pressure suggests a space-occupying lesion or cerebral oedema.
Protein	< 0.4 g/l	Raised protein is common to many neurological diseases and is non-specific.
White cells	< 5 per mm^3 No polymorphs, mononuclear cells only	White cells in the CSF suggest inflammation in the meninges. Polymorphonuclear cells suggest a pyogenic infection. Viral encephalitis produces mainly lymphocytes in the CSF. A slight pleocytosis can be present in other conditions, including tumours, infarction, carcinomatous malignancy and multiple sclerosis (MS).
Protein electrophoresis (oligoclonal bands)	Suggests an inflammatory disorder. A matched serum sample will determine whether the bands are of CNS origin. Found in MS, sarcoid, systemic lupus erythematosus (SLE) and cerebral vasculitis.	
Glucose	> 0.6 × blood glucose	A lowered CSF glucose (< 60% of plasma glucose) suggests a bacterial meningitis.
Specific brain proteins	These are generally protein components of nerve and glial cells in the brain that are released when the brain is damaged. In general, they are raised in proportion to the rate of progression of the disease.	
14-3-3	Raised levels are particularly associated with CJD (Hsich et al, 1996), although this is not specific to CJD and may be seen in herpes encephalitis.	

Table 3
Continued

Parameter	Normal finding
Neurone-specific enolase	A neuronal protein, which, when raised, suggests neurodegeneration and supports a diagnosis of a degenerative dementia.
S100β	An astrocytic protein, and raised levels may be associated with astrocytosis, such as in FTD (Green et al, 1997).
Tau	Hyperphosphorylated tau protein is the major constituent of the paired helical filaments forming neurofibrillary tangles in AD. The demonstration of raised CSF tau has a sensitivity of approximately 77% and a specificity of approximately 63% in differentiating AD patients from normal controls. However, tau is also raised in other neurodegenerative diseases associated with tau deposition.

Diagnostic genetic testing

Advances in the molecular genetics of the dementias are providing an increasing range of possible mutations that can be tested for. The implications of a positive test for a specific genetic mutations are much wider than simply confirming a diagnosis. The most obvious will be that the patient's offspring will be at 50% risk of carrying the mutation and thus developing the disease. Testing should be carried out only after genetic counselling of the patient and family. It would rarely be appropriate to carry out blanket screening for genetic mutations.

For at-risk family members who are requesting predictive genetic testing, genetic counselling may be carried out in a specialist genetics clinic following the protocol devised for Huntington's disease (Sadovnick and Lovestone, 1996), although it is necessary to have determined the family-specific mutation in an affected individual first.

Table 4 summarises the genetic mutations relevant to patients with dementia, with suggested indications for considering the test.

Table 4
Genetic mutations and indications of relevance to patients with dementia.

Gene	Indication	Comments
Huntington	Suspected Huntington's disease	
Prion	Suspected CJD, particularly where there is a family history of young onset, rapidly progressive or atypical dementia	A range of point mutations and pathogenic repeat insertions in the human prion protein gene have been identified.
Presenilin-1 and -2	Suspected AD with age at onset 32–64 years, usually with a positive family history	Point mutations and pathogenic deletions have been identified in the presenilin-1 gene on chromosome 14 and the presenilin-2 gene on chromosome 1, By comparison, only a small number of mutations in the APP gene on chromosome 21 have been found, suggesting that this is a very rare cause of AD. Current evidence suggests that random screening of AD patients is very unlikely to identify mutations, and testing should be reserved for those where there is a strong family history of AD.
APP	Suspected AD with a family history, young onset and negative PS-1 mutation testing	
Tau	Suspected familial frontotemporal dementia	Mutations have recently been identified in the tau gene on chromosome 17. The prevalence of these mutations in the FTD patient population is, as yet, unknown. Testing should probably be reserved for patients with a family history.

Table 4
Continued

Gene	Indication	Comments
Notch 3	Suspected familial vascular dementia	Mutations in the *notch 3* gene result in a familial vascular dementia termed Cerebral Autosomal Dominant Angiography with Subcortical Infarcts and Leukoencephalopathy (CADASIL). Testing should be considered for younger patients with vascular dementia and a strong family history.
Apolipoprotein E4 (ApoE4)	Not indicated for clinical use	ApoE4 is a risk factor for developing AD. Inheriting one E4 allele increases the risk of developing AD by four times. However, it is not causative of the disease, and having even two copies of the E4 allele does not necessarily result in the disease. In established disease it is not diagnostic, and pre-symptomatically it is not predictive, therefore the test has no place in current clinical practice.

Biopsy

Muscle biopsy

Muscle biopsy can be a useful investigation in suspected mitochondrial disorders ('ragged-red' skeletal muscle fibres), CADASIL and ceroid lipo-fuscinosis (Kuf's disease).

Tonsillar biopsy

The lymphoreticular tissue in the tonsils has been shown to stain for abnormal prion protein in variant CJD (vCJD). A positive tonsillar biopsy can confirm diagnosis and avoids the need for more invasive cerebral biopsy in cases of suspected vCJD (Hill et al, 1999).

Cerebral biopsy

Ultimately, in a very small number of patients it is necessary to carry out a cerebral biopsy to provide a histological diagnosis. The biopsy specimen is usually taken from the non-dominant frontal lobe but may be guided by areas of change (e.g. inflammation) seen on MRI. The indications for cerebral biopsy are relatively younger patients (although this is not absolute) with atypical and/or rapidly progressive dementia, particularly where an inflammatory cause is suspected. A common reason for biopsy is in suspected cerebral vasculitis where intervention with steroids may be curative. It is critically important that the biopsy is carried out by an experienced neurosurgeon and includes a full-thickness cortical sample to include white matter and pia mater.

Diagnosis

Introduction

We have divided diagnosis in dementia into three sections. The first section covers the major causes of dementia, where, for each disease we have covered the epidemiology, a clinical description, summarised diagnostic criteria and supporting investigations. The second section covers less common causes of dementia that are likely to be seen in clinical practice, while the final section covers rare causes of dementia that nevertheless need to be considered as more common causes are ruled out. The flow-chart presented in **Figure 8** summarises some clinical pointers that can assist the process of differential diagnosis, particularly if neuroimaging is available.

Figure 8
A summary of clinical pointers assisting in the differential diagnosis of dementia.

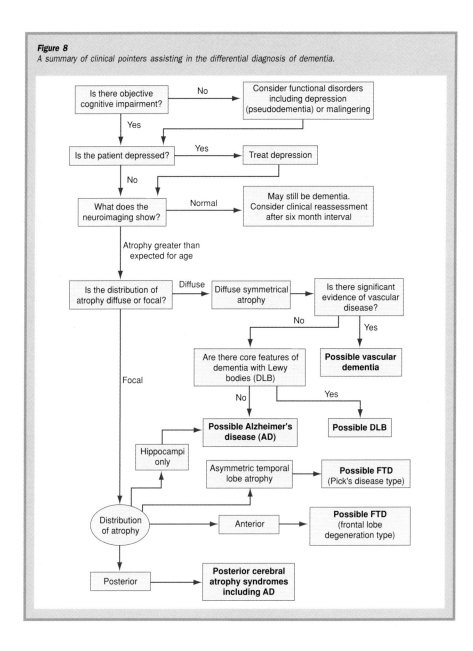

The major causes of dementia

Alzheimer's disease

Alzheimer's disease (AD) is strictly a neuropathological diagnosis determined by the presence of neurofibrillary tangles and senile plaques in the brain of a patient with dementia (Gearing et al, 1995). The disease frequently starts with memory impairment, but is invariably followed by a progressive global cognitive impairment. General neurological examination is often normal early in the disease. Structural neuroimaging may also be normal early in the disease, but cerebral atrophy, particularly of the medial temporal lobe structures, is apparent as the disease progresses (Rossor, 1993).

Epidemiology

Figure 9 illustrates the prevalence of AD in the general population according to age.

Relevant investigations in Alzheimer's disease

History	The history will usually be of an insidious onset, often starting with memory deficits. The decline is slow and progressive with disorientation and increasing dependence upon carers. Depression is a common feature, and seizures may occur later in the illness. Neurological signs, seizures early in the disease, preserved memory and step-wise or rapid progression would all be against a diagnosis of AD
Neuropsychology	Typically progressive episodic memory impairment is an early sign, with global cognitive deficits developing as the disease progresses. Isolated preservation of neuropsychological abilities, particularly later in the disease, would be against a diagnosis of AD.
Neuroimaging	CT or MRI may be reported as normal early in the disease. Atrophy of medial temporal lobe structures (which includes the hippocampus) is usually seen with more generalised atrophy as the disease progresses. Preservation of medial temporal lobe structures (the hippocampus), multiple infarcts, significant white-matter signal change (more than periventricular) and focal or asymmetrical atrophy would be against a diagnosis of pure AD.
Other tests	A routine blood screen is likely to be normal. There are no specific diagnostic tests.

Diagnostic criteria – DSM-IV

A DSM-IV (American Psychiatric Association, 1994) diagnosis of AD requires the patient to have developed deficits in multiple domains of cognitive function, which consist of:

• Memory impairment

Plus one or more impairments in the domains:

• Language (aphasia)
• Motor activities (apraxia)
• Visual perception (agnosia)
• Executive functioning (frontal lobe function).

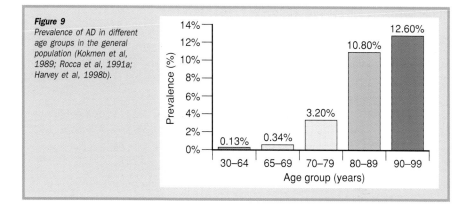

Figure 9
Prevalence of AD in different age groups in the general population (Kokmen et al, 1989; Rocca et al, 1991a; Harvey et al, 1998b).

Furthermore these deficits should be significant enough to impair social and/or occupational function. The development of these symptoms should have been gradual, progressive and not associated with other CNS diseases, systemic disorders known to cause cognitive impairment, or substance abuse. The deficits should not occur exclusively during a delirium, and should not be better accounted for by any other DMS-IV diagnosis, for example a major depressive disorder.

Vascular dementia

Neuropathologically, vascular dementia (VaD) includes cases of dementia resulting from ischaemic and haemorrhagic brain lesions, and from ischaemic–hypoxic damage such as occurs following cardiac arrest. These pathological changes result from a range of underlying aetiologies complicating accurate diagnosis in life. Diagnosis is also complicated by the uncertainty of ascertaining the temporal relationship between cerebral insults such as strokes, and the onset of the dementia.

In 1993, a work group of the National Institute of Neurological Disorders and Stroke (NINDS) and the Association Internationale pour la Recherche et l'Enseignement en Neurosciences (AIREN) reported on a workshop held to discuss diagnostic criteria for research in VaD (Roman et al, 1993). They recognised the difficulties inherent in the diagnosis, and classified VaD syndromes as follows:

- Small vessel disease with dementia
- Multi-infarct dementia
- Strategic single-infarct dementia
- Hypoperfusion
- Haemorrhagic dementia
- Other mechanisms.

Moreover, cerebrovascular disease is common in the elderly and is likely to be a complicating component in many cases of AD.

Epidemiology

Figure 10 illustrates the prevalence of VaD in the general population according to age.

Diagnostic criteria

Diagnostic criteria for VaD are less well developed (Verhey et al, 1996) and there is no firm consensus on the most appropriate criteria to use for clinical practice (Antuono et al, 1997).

DSM-IV criteria (American Psychiatric Association, 1994) are very similar to the criteria for AD, but require the presence of focal neurological symptoms, or neuroimaging signs of multiple infarctions in the cortex. The ICD-10 criteria require a history of transient ischaemic attacks, or a succession of small strokes. The importance of demonstrating the presence of vascular risk factors is recognised, together with the findings of focal neurological signs and symptoms, and neuroimaging confirmation of vascular lesions (World Health Organisation, 1992).

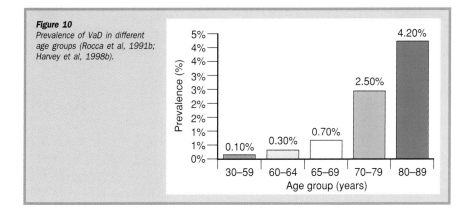

Figure 10
Prevalence of VaD in different age groups (Rocca et al, 1991b; Harvey et al, 1998b).

Relevant investigations in vascular dementia

History	The history is more often of an abrupt onset with a stepwise deterioration. Eliciting the presence of vascular risk factors, such as hypertension, smoking, cardiovascular disease, diabetes and hypercholesterolaemia are important, particularly since managing these risk factors may reduce the rate of progression of the disease.
Examination	Focal neurological, pyramidal or extrapyramidal signs may be present. A characteristic broad-based, small-stepping gait (*marche à petit pas*) may be present. Examination of the cardiovascular system is important in the evaluation of risk factors for VaD.
Neuropsychology	Classically, aphasia visuoperceptual and visuospatial deficits are associated with cortical vascular lesions. The deficits may be focal, and memory, although affected, may be less impaired relative to other deficits.
Neuroimaging	CT or MRI is critical in making a diagnosis of VaD. MRI in particular is helpful in demonstrating infarcts and white-matter lesions. MR angiography or doppler ultrasound may demonstrate surgically amenable carotid stenosis.
Other tests	In addition to a routine screen, initial investigation of suspected VaD should include plasma lipids, and a full cardiovascular work-up including ECG and echocardiogram. Investigations are made primarily to identify or exclude treatable risk factors and causes for emboli. Muscle biopsy and testing for *notch 3* mutations may be helpful in the diagnosis of CADASIL.

Dementia with Lewy bodies

The neuropathological hallmark of dementia with Lewy bodies (DLB) is the finding of numerous eosinophilic inclusions (Lewy Bodies) in cortical neurones of a patient with dementia. Rarely, Lewy bodies are the only pathological changes present, more commonly there are also Alzheimer-type senile plaques. Neurofibrillary tangles are usually rare or absent.

Relevant investigations in dementia with Lewy bodies

History	The history should cover psychiatric symptoms, particularly visual hallucinations. Direct questioning of the caregiver may be needed to elicit such symptoms, along with evidence of fluctuation in cognition. Some patients have a dramatic psychiatric presentation to their illness.
Examination	Motor signs of Parkinsonism are an important component of the diagnosis, although their absence does not exclude DLB. Some patients also develop myoclonus.
Neuropsychology	Visuospatial, visuoperceptual and frontal deficits are common in DLB. The memory impairment, particularly early in the disease may be proportionally less than the deficits in other domains.
Neuroimaging	Usually very similar to AD with generalised cortical atrophy that involves the medial temporal lobe structures. Prominent white-matter change and numerous infarcts are more suggestive of a vascular dementia that may have a similar presentation.
Other tests	For patients with motor features of Parkinsonism an L-DOPA challenge will demonstrate whether these symptoms are amenable to treatment, but can exacerbate the hallucinations and cognitive impairment.

DLB is characterised by progressive cognitive decline particularly affecting attention, frontal subcortical skills and visuo-perceptual abilities. The cognitive impairment often fluctuates and there may be visual hallucinations and motor features of Parkinsonism. In addition, there may be falls, syncopal episodes, transient disturbances of consciousness, neuroleptic sensitivity, delusions and hallucinations in other modalities. It is not unusual for patients with DLB to suffer disturbed sleep, nightmares and abnormal behaviour at night.

Epidemiology

There is relatively little epidemiological data available for DLB. Post-mortem series suggest that up to 20% of dementia in elderly patients may be the result of DLB (McKeith et al, 1994). DLB in younger patients may be less common; in a recent epidemiological study of pre-senile dementia, a clinical diagnosis of DLB was made in 3% of patients (Harvey et al, 1998b).

Diagnostic criteria

The consensus criteria for DLB (McKeith et al, 1996) require evidence of progressive cognitive decline of sufficient magnitude to interfere with normal social or occupational function. Prominent memory impairment may not occur in the early stages but is evident with progression of the disease. Deficits on tests of attention and of frontal subcortical skills and visuo-spatial ability may be especially prominent. Two of the following three core features are essential for a diagnosis of probable DLB: fluctuating cognition; visual hallucinations; motor features of Parkinsonism. Features supporting the diagnosis include: repeated falls; syncope; transient disturbances of consciousness; neuroleptic sensitivity; systemised delusions; and hallucinations in other modalities.

Frontotemporal dementia

Frontotemporal dementia (FTD) describes a clinical syndrome of behav-ioural disorder and progressive cogni-tive decline associated with frontotem-poral cerebral atrophy (Gustafson, 1987; The Lund and Manchester Groups, 1994), usually beginning before the age of 65 years. The syndrome has three main pathological substrates: in the frontal lobe degenera-tion type nerve cell loss and spongi-form change is seen; in the Pick's disease type, swollen or 'ballooned' neurones (Pick cells) and intraneuronal tau-positive inclusion bodies (Pick bodies) are present; and in the third variant of the disease, spinal motor neurone degeneration occurs in associa-tion with frontal lobe degeneration type pathology, and motor neurone disease type inclusions (Neary et al, 1993).

The core clinical features of these patients are the insidious onset of a selective loss of cognitive abilities, namely language and/or frontal execu-tive function, with the relative preser-vation in other domains such as episodic memory, orientation and visuoperceptual function. Personal and social awareness is lost early, and the disease is associated with disinhibition, mental rigidity and inflexibility in association with maintained general independence.

Relevant investigations in frontotemporal dementia

History	The history is commonly of a very insidious onset of the disease with either subtle language or personality changes. The focal nature of the disease provides a key diagnostic feature, that of preserved areas of ability. Patients are rarely disorientated and can often go out independently even late in the illness. Probing for preserved abilities is important when taking the history. Dietary changes in terms of over-eating, rigidity in the diet and a preference for sweet food is common.
Examination	The neurological examination should include primitive reflexes, which appear early in the disease, the demonstration of apraxia, and a careful examination for muscle fasciculation, suggesting anterior horn cell disease, seen most commonly in the deltoid muscles. The presence of utilisation behaviour may be a dramatic demonstration of frontal dysfunction.
Neuropsychology	A number of characteristic patterns of neuropsychological deficits may be seen in FTD. An important diagnostic feature is the demonstration of preserved visuoperceptual and visuospatial abilities. Particular patterns of deficits include progressive aphasia, semantic memory impairment and frontal deficits. A pattern of asymmetrical deficits or progressive focal deficits in the frontal and/or temporal lobes with selective preservation of more posterior function is highly supportive of a diagnosis of FTD.
Neuroimaging	CT, or ideally MRI, is an important diagnostic investigation. Focal and/or asymmetrical atrophy affecting frontal and/or temporal lobe structures (best seen on coronal slices) is highly supportive of the diagnosis.
Other tests	Patients with muscle fasciculation should have an EMG. An EEG that is normal in the presence of significant objective frontotemporal cognitive impairment supports a diagnosis of FTD.

Epidemiology

Very little is known of the epidemiology of FTD. A recent study suggests that it may account for up to 18% of dementia in people under the age of 65 years (Harvey et al, 1998b).

Alcohol-related dementia

Alcohol-related dementia (ARD) refers to patients with a history of chronic alcohol abuse, presenting with cognitive impairments and fulfilling the criteria for dementia. As with primary degenerative dementias, the deficits progress with continued drinking, however, there is evidence to suggest that they may become static or even regress if abstinence is attained (Tuck et al, 1984). In addition to general ARD, there are a number of specific syndromes related to alcohol-induced brain damage: Wernicke–Korsakoff syndrome (thiamine deficiency); Marchiafava–Bignami disease; pellagrous encephalopathy (niacin deficiency); and acquired hepatocerebral degeneration (shunting of portal blood to the systemic circulation) (Victor, 1994).

Patients have deficits of memory function, speed and attention, visuo-perceptual function and particularly frontal lobe (executive) function (Grant, 1987; Pohl, 1987). Neuro-psychological deficits are usually mild to moderate and show slow, but never complete, recovery with abstinence. The presence of frontal lobe deficits seems to predict a poor outcome as abstinence is difficult to maintain,

resulting in a chronic downwards spiral (Gurling et al, 1986; Goldman, 1990). Neuroimaging studies consistently show cerebral atrophy in 50–70% of chronic alcoholics, with cortical shrinkage and ventricular enlargement, particularly affecting the frontal lobes (Gurling et al, 1986; Smith and Atkinson, 1995; Lishman, 1997).

Epidemiology

Few studies have attempted to measure the prevalence of an alcoholic dementia syndrome. Copeland et al (1992), in a study based on 1070 people over the age of 65 years living in Liverpool, found a prevalence of 0.3% for alcohol-related dementia. Surveys of alcoholics attending for treatment suggest that up to 50% of those over the age of 45 years with a lengthy drinking history will have evidence of cognitive impairment (Edwards, 1982). In surveys of patients being investigated as inpatients for dementia by psychiatrists, up to 10% have been found to have alcohol as the most likely contributing cause (Lishman, 1997).

Diagnostic criteria

The DSM-IV criteria for alcohol-induced persisting dementia (AIPD) require the criteria for dementia with evidence from the history, physical examination or inves- tigations that the deficits are aetiologically related to the persisting effects of alcohol.

Relevant investigations in alcohol-related dementia

History	The history should document the symptoms of dementia and history of alcohol abuse, with an attempt to link the two. It is important to establish current alcohol consumption and social situation to plan appropriate management.
Examination	Examination should focus on identifying physical stigmata of alcohol abuse and liver disease.
Neuropsychology	The neuropsychological examination may show a picture of global cognitive impairment, however, prominent frontal deficits would support the diagnosis.
Neuroimaging	CT or MRI are likely to show global atrophy. There may also be evidence or previous head trauma or intracranial bleeding.

Less common causes of dementia

Prion diseases

The prion diseases are lethal, degenerative brain diseases arising from abnormal protein folding of a normal cellular prion protein (PrP^c) to create a pathological isoform (PrP^{sc}). The change in protein folding may occur rarely as a spontaneous event (sporadic disease), or as a result of a mutation in the prion protein gene (familial), or can be induced in the normal protein by exposure to the abnormal isoform (transmissible). In humans, prion disease may be familial, sporadic, iatrogenic or transmissible (**see Table 5**). Iatrogenic prion diseases include the transmission of the disease through the use of pooled human pituitary-derived growth hormone, cadaveric corneal and dura mater grafts, and the use of prion-contaminated neurosurgical and electrophysiological instruments. Additional transmissible forms of the disease include Kuru, due to endocannibalism, which is now disappearing, and variant CJD (vCJD), believed to be transmitted from bovine spongiform

Table 5
Human prion disease (after Collinge, 1997).

Type	Clinical syndrome	Aetiology
Acquired	Kuru	Cannibalism
	Iatrogenic CJD	Accidental inoculation with human prions (pooled cadaveric growth hormone, corneal transplants, cadaveric dura mater grafts, neurosurgical instruments)
	Variant CJD	Dietary or environmental exposure to pathogenic bovine prion protein. Currently only seen in the UK
Sporadic	CJD	Spontaneous conversion of normal to pathogenic prion protein
	Atypical CJD	
Familial	Familial CJD	Autosomal dominant prion protein gene mutations. These may produce a range of phenotypes, which have previously been given different names including: fatal familial insomnia (FFI) and Gerstmann–Straussler–Scheinker disease (GSS).

encephalopathy (BSE). Prion diseases affect approximately 1 person per million world-wide (Collinge, 1997).

Diagnosis is based upon the history and characteristic clinical features, including rapid progression with additional relatively specific neurological features, which commonly include myoclonus. Characteristic EEG changes are seen in up to 70% of cases of sporadic CJD. A tonsillar biopsy that is positive for prion protein may be diagnostic in vCJD. Variant CJD has only been recently seen in the UK and, so far, affects younger adults (typically aged 20 to 40 years), unlike classical CJD where the mean age at onset is around 65 years. The presentation is often of behavioural change followed by complaints of peripheral parasthesiae and progressive ataxia before, or simultaneous with, cognitive decline. The course of the disease is rapid, with expected survival being around 2 years. It is slightly less catastrophic than classical CJD, where median survival is around only 1 year. EEG changes may not be present in early vCJD.

Corticobasal degeneration

Corticobasal degeneration (CBD) is a rare form of dementia with clinical features that are a combination of cognitive impairment and asymmetrical motor symptoms. The neuropathological diagnosis is based macroscopically on the finding of frontoparietal neuronal loss and gliosis, which is often asymmetrical. Microscopically there are cortical ballooned neurones, degeneration of the substantia nigra and variable involvement of the subcortical nuclei, including the basal ganglia. The heterogeneity of the clinical presentation, with initial symptoms of either cognitive or motor symptoms, result in some patients being referred to neurologists or geriatricians interested in movement disorders, while others are referred to neurologists or psychiatrists interested in dementia.

In a recent review of consecutive autopsy diagnosed cases, CBD was usually only one of several differential diagnoses (Schneider et al, 1997).

Other clinical diagnoses included Parkinson's disease, VaD, atypical AD, MND, Pick's disease and DLB. This heterogeneity is also present neuropathologically with many cases having neuropathological features of other degenerative dementias, as well as CBD. Despite this heterogeneity of clinical diagnosis and neuropathology, the clinical presentations are fairly constant. Most cases with asymmetrical motor symptoms, often described as a stiff hand or arm, or difficulty with writing. Other patients present with cognitive impairment but later develop this asymmetrical apraxia. Nearly all cases have extrapyramidal symptoms in the form of combinations of brady-kinesia, 'alien limb', rigidity, tremor and postural instability; often inviting a diagnosis of Parkinson's disease.

Huntington's disease

Huntington's disease (HD) is a hereditary progressive neurological disease characterised by a triad of clinical features: motor symptoms; cognitive impairment; and psychiatric disturbance. The motor features include abnormalities of both voluntary movement (e.g. clumsiness, brady-kinesia, rigidity, gait disturbance, dysarthria, dysphagia and saccadic eye movements) and involuntary movement (e.g. chorea, dystonia, athetosis, motor restlessness and myoclonus). The prominence of the chorea usually results in referral to neurologists with an interest in movement disorders rather than to dementia or memory clinics. The cognitive deficits relate to impairment of memory, calculation, verbal fluency, visuospatial ability and frontal executive skills. By contrast, aphasia, apraxia and agnosia are uncommon in HD. Psychiatrically, patients commonly develop depression with a high incidence of suicide. Patients may also become irritable and disinhibited, but are rarely psychotic. Diagnosis is based upon the history and examination, particularly in the presence of a family history. Diagnosis can be confirmed by genetic testing (Jones et al, 1997; Chui, 1994).

Progressive supranuclear palsy

Progressive supranuclear palsy (PSP; also referred to as Steele–Richardson–Osliewski Syndrome) is a disease associated with neurodegeneration of the pons, midbrain, dentate and subthalamic nuclei, globus pallidus and nucleus basalis. Histologically, the pathological hallmarks of the disease are neurofibril-

lary tangles (ultrastructurally distinct from Alzheimer's tangles) and gloisis in the absence of senile plaques. Clinically, the syndrome is quite diverse, with a variable age at onset, and with a substantial overlap with other cognitive and movement disorders. The key features in the diagnosis are early downward gaze palsy, symmetrical Parkinsonism with ataxia, rigidity, disequilibrium (instability), early falling and progressive dementia. Features that support the diagnosis include symmetrical motor symptoms, early gait disturbance, frequent and early falls, an erect posture, late loss of arm swing and a 'surprised' facial expression with loss of blinking. Features against PSP include visual hallucinations (which suggest DLB), 'alien limb' phenomena (which suggest CBD) and autonomic failure (which suggests multi system atrophy MSA) (Sagar, 1998).

Dementia in Parkinson's disease

Parkinson's disease (PD) is characterised pathologically by the presence of Lewy bodies in the substantia nigra and other brain stem nuclei. Approximately one-third of PD patients develop dementia as the disease progresses, probably as Lewy bodies spread from the brain stem to the cortex, although other mechanisms have also been suggested. The clinical features of dementia in PD are, however, very similar to those of patients with DLB. The most common presentation is increasing mental inflexibility in a patient with PD, followed by defects of executive function, marked fluctuation and, in many cases, visual hallucinations. The hallucinations are often exacerbated by anticholinergic and dopamine agonist medications. Management is very similar to DLB, and much of the management is often balancing the need to treat the motor symptoms of PD, while minimising the side-effects of the treatments in terms of worsened cognition and neuro-psychiatric features. Depression is common in this condition and should be rigorously identified and treated.

HIV/AIDS dementia

As many as one-third of patients with the acquired immunodeficiency syndrome (AIDS) eventually develop dementia (Lipton, 1997). HIV dementia is a pervasive neurological disorder resulting in global cognitive impairment, progressive weakness and frequent psychiatric symptoms, including depression, anxiety and mania. The disease is most commonly associated with the late manifestations of AIDS, and the patient will usually have evidence of severe immunosuppression. With recent advances in therapy, however, the prevalence of HIV/AIDS dementia may be diminishing. Neuroimaging is extremely important in diagnosis and may show cerebral atrophy, white-matter lesions or evidence of other CNS manifestations of AIDS, such as toxoplasmosis or cryptosporidiosis.

Rare causes of dementia

There are more than 200 diseases that can be associated with progressive cognitive impairment and dementia. Many are exceptionally rare, while others have very specific and characteristic physical signs and pathophysiological features. **Table 6** summarises some of the rare causes of dementia that can present significant diagnostic challenges. Further details on rarer causes of dementia can be found in Rossor (1999).

Table 6 *Some of the rarer causes of dementia.*

Disease	Pathophysiology	Characteristic features and diagnostic tests
Normal-pressure hydrocephalus	The causes of normal-pressure hydrocephalus include trauma, subarachnoid haemorrhage, and meningitis but, in some cases, the condition may be idiopathic.	The cognitive impairment shows a psychomotor slowing with prominent subcortical features. Patients with a known cause and a short history, and those in whom imaging shows small cortical sulci and peri-ventricular lucencies, i.e. those in whom an additional degenerative dementia is unlikely, respond best to shunting with respect to the cognitive impairment.
Progressive subcortical gliosis	A disease characterised by astrocytosis throughout the cortex associated with cerebral atrophy. The cause is unknown.	Usually presents with a slowly progressive dementia without other prominent neurological features. Very few cases have been described, although a long duration of disease (up to 20 years) may be characteristic. The disease may mimic other rare forms of dementia, such as PSP.
Cerebral vasculitis	An inflammatory disorder of cerebral vessels that may be a primary disorder (Wegener's granulomatosis, microscopic polyangitis, temporal arteritis), or secondary to other systemic diseases (collagen vascular or rheumatological disorders, malignancy, drugs and infections).	The presentation may be with either an acute or subacute encephalopathy, a syndrome with similarities to MS (MS-Plus), or with features of a rapidly progressive space-occupying lesion (Scolding et al, 1997). An elevated ESR or CRP should lead to suspicion. MRI is abnormal in the majority of patients. Vasculitis may be visible on ophthalmological examination with video microscopy and low-dose fluorescein angiography. Oligoclonal bands may be present in the CSF. A cerebral biopsy is diagnostic. The potential treatability of this condition is the major reason for invasive investigation. Treatment with steroids, in some cases augmented with immunosuppression, may be dramatically effective.
Dementia in multiple sclerosis	Up to 40% of community-resident MS patients have significant cognitive impairment.	Since MS is a disease of white matter, the dementia associated with MS most commonly has subcortical features. Cognitive function declines as the disease progresses and remains static when the disease is static. The cognitive impairment is readily detected on neuropsychological testing.

Disease	Pathophysiology	Characteristic features and diagnostic tests
Wilson's disease	A disorder of copper metabolism transmitted as an autosomal recessive trait. Found in 3 per 100 000 people.	Commonly presents with psychiatric symptoms of all types. It also presents rarely as a dementia. Neurological manifestations, such as tremor, dystonia and dysarthria are common. Kayser–Fleischer rings demonstrated in the cornea by slit-lamp examination are diagnostic. Diagnosis can also be confirmed by finding a low serum copper and caeruloplasmin, with an elevated urinary copper excretion.
Metachromatic leukodystrophy	A disorder of myelin metabolism due to lack of arylsulphatase A enzyme results in accumulation of sulpha-tides, which stain with a meta-chromatic appearance. It is an auto-somal recessively inherited disorder.	This is the adult variant of the disease that may present from the mid-teens to mid-70s, with peripheral neuropathy, cognitive impairment and behavioural change. In particular, there are often frontal lobe deficits and personality changes. Spasticity, emotional lability and involuntary movements often accompany the dementia. The diagnosis is made by demonstrating reduced arylsulphatase activity in white blood cells. Metachromatic lipid material may also be seen in samples obtained from centrifuged urine or CSF.
Niemann–Pick disease type C	Associated with accumulation of sphingomyelin and other lipids in the liver, spleen and bone marrow. The type C variant presents at any time from infancy to adulthood, with neurological symptoms and hepatosplenomegaly.	The neurological signs of the disorder are characteristic with hepatosplenomegaly, ataxia, dementia, dystonia and supranuclear ophthalmoplegia. The adult-onset disorder progresses more slowly, but can be associated with psychosis. Diagnosis can be made on bone marrow examination, which shows 'foam' cells. Elevated levels of sphingomyelin, cholesterol or glycolipids can also be demonstrated in liver biopsy samples.
Kuf's disease	A rare lysosomal storage disease, part of a group of disease termed neuroanal ceroid lipofuscinoses. The childhood-onset forms are known as Batten's disease. The late-onset form typically starts around 30 years of age.	Onset is usually with dementia, epilepsy, dysarthria, facial dyskinesia and cerebellar signs. There are also commonly personality and behavioural changes, including psychosis. The seizures usually become intractable. Definitive diagnosis is by demonstrating characteristic granular deposits on electron microscopy of skin or cerebral biopsy material.

Continued overleaf

Table 6 *Some of the rarer causes of dementia (continued)*

Disease	Pathophysiology	Characteristic features and diagnostic tests
Other storage diseases	A range of other storage diseases can present with dementia in adult life. They are commonly recessively inherited with a presentation in young adult life.	
Whipple's disease	A rare multi-system disorder most commonly presenting in middle-aged men.	CNS symptoms occur in 40% of cases. Care systemic features include malabsorption weight loss, pyrexia, polyarthralgia and lymphadenopathy. CSF examination shows a raised protein and the presence of oligoclonal bands. PAS-positive cells may be present in the CSF. Diagnosis is by demonstrating PAS-positive deposits within macrophages, obtained either from a jejunal or cerebral biopsy. Antibiotic therapy may halt the disease in some cases.
Mitochondrial diseases (Suomalainen, 1997)	There have been rapid advances in our understanding of mitochondrial function and the identification of specific diseases. A number of these involve cognitive impairment. One of the better characterised mitochondrial syndromes associated with dementia is MELAS (mitochondrial encephalomyopathy, lactic acidosis and stroke-like episodes). In its most common form, it results in stroke-like episodes beginning before the age of 40, encephalopathy associated with seizures and dementia, lactic acidosis and the finding of ragged-red fibres on muscle biopsy. A range of mutations in the mtDNA result in MELAS and other encephalomyopathies.	The diagnosis of mitochondrial diseases is not easy. In the family history there may be evidence of material inheritance, although the variability, both in the phenotype and severity of the disease may make this difficult to detect. 'Soft' clinical signs in both the patient and relatives, such as headaches, deafness, short stature, ophthalmoplegia and diabetes, may also gives clues to the involvement of mitochondrial defects. The pathological hallmarks of mitochondrial diseases are the finding of ragged-red fibres in a muscle biopsy specimen. The ragged-red appearance is due to the over-production of non-functional mitochondria, which are also enlarged, distorted and contain abnormal inclusions. Biochemical analysis of the affected tissue may reveal a specific defect or combination of defects in the respiratory chain enzymes.

Management

Support

Providing support for the patient, family and carers is central to delivering the highest quality of care in dementia. Support should be made available from the initial presentation with the disease, through the period of diagnosis, to entry into institutional care, and for the family even after the affected person has died.

Any appropriately trained member of staff can deliver basic support to carers and families; however, the specialist nurse is often the most appropriate person to take the lead in developing and delivering care and support to the patient and their family.

The following sections cover the broad areas of support that can be built up into an effective framework of care.

Advice and information

Both the patient and the carer should have access to advice and information from the earliest stages of the disease. Initially there is likely to be a need for information and reassurance about the process of diagnosis and the tests that are being proposed. Most people will not understand terms such as dementia, Alzheimer's disease, MRI scan etc. and will need simple explanations about what is going on.

Once a diagnosis has been made it is important that the patient and family is given this news in a sensitive and supportive way. It is usually the doctor's role to pass on the diagnosis, however, it is helpful if the patient and family can then have the opportunity to discuss the diagnosis and its implications with an experienced nurse or other member of the team. Basic information about the range of diseases that cause dementia are needed. Families will almost always want to know about prognosis and what will happen as the disease progresses, and in some circumstances a more detailed diagnosis will need to be given to the carer than the patient. While it is important to stress that the course for a particular patient cannot be predicted, it is sensible to prepare, gently and sensitively, the patient and family for what will happen in the future. Patients and carers can sometimes fail to comprehend the progressive natures of the dementias.

As the disease progresses more information can be given. The onset of behavioural problems, other symptoms such as incontinence, and the time when decisions are being made about long-term care are particular times when information about where to get help and advice on the problems are needed.

After the patient has died, and where a post-mortem has been carried out to confirm the diagnosis, families will often benefit from the opportunity to discuss the results and the final diagnosis, particularly if it differs from the clinical diagnosis made in life.

Medical care and specialists

For those patients initially seen by a neurologist or general physician, consideration should be given to referring the patient to an old-age psychiatrist or geriatrician who may have better access to appropriate support services. Simialrly, psychiatrists and old-age psychiatrists assessing a patient with atypical neurological signs should seek the advice of a neurologist.

Inevitably, while the majority of patients with dementia are cared for by general practitioners, knowledge of and access to multidisciplinary community support services, as well as secondary care services is critical to delivering the most effective care.

Driving

It is vital to ask about driving in every case of dementia. Patients with significant cognitive impairment or a diagnosis of dementia are legally required to inform the driving licence authorities and their motor insurers of their medical problems. The licensing authorities' medical examiner will then make a decision on whether to rescind the license based upon medical reports.

If a patient with dementia is found to be still driving, it is helpful to discuss the issue with the carer, and particularly to ask the carer and other family members whether they feel safe in the car with the patient driving. If they report feeling safe in the car, and the patient's cognitive impairments are not severe, then it is probably safe to allow them to continue to drive until the licensing authorities make a decision. If, however, the family reports feeling unsafe, or report potentially dangerous incidents then the patient should be advised to stop driving immediately, and not to drive until the licensing

authority have made their decision, which will inevitably be to take away the license. Visuoperceptual and visuospatial impairments, dyspraxia and frontal syndromes can give rise to more problematic driving decisions than memory or language impairment.

Benefits and finances

Ensuring that the patient and carer have adequate financial support is an important practical way that help can be provided. If the patient is still working or is on sick leave then they will need to take professional advice regarding pension provisions. Early or hasty retirement on medical grounds may adversely affect long-term pension rights.

Encouraging the patient and carer to sign an **Enduring Power of Attorney** early in the illness can be vital in ensuring that the patient's finances are managed appropriately once the disease has progressed to the point where they are no longer able to manage them themselves.

In the UK, patients under the age of 65 years should be encouraged to apply for **Disability Living Allowance** while patients above retirement age should apply for **Attendance Allowance** to provide financial support for their care.

Assistance is often needed with applications, as the information required by the application forms will often focus on physical disability rather than cognitive impairment. Involving a clinic nurse with experience in helping families complete the forms can be very valuable.

Medic-alert bracelet

Encouraging the patient to wear a medical identification bracelet (Medic-Alert) should ensure that they receive rapid and appropriate medical or social care, for example if they wander and become displaced from their carer or family.

Voluntary services

There are now many charities supporting patients with dementia and their families. It is important to put sufferers and carers in touch with support and information as early as possible in the illness. Appendix 1 lists the names and addresses of the major voluntary organisations and support services; in most cases there will be local branches and support groups.

Social services

Social Services are the main route of access to community- and home-based care for patients with dementia and their carers. Referral to Social Services should be considered early in the illness, even if services are not obviously immediately needed. An early comprehensive community care assessment can facilitate obtaining benefits, and the transition to day care and eventual residential care may be easier as the disease progresses.

Social Services provide access to the home-based and community-based services, which are summarised below:

- Community-based services
    - Information, support and referral services
    - Support groups
    - Community transport
    - Case management
    - Advocacy services
    - Day centres
    - Respite care
    - Residential care
- Home-based services
    - Outreach services
    - Sitting services
    - Domiciliary care and home nursing

- Meals on wheels
- Careline (emergency telephone).

Not every area will provide all of these facilities, but often access to any of these types of support can only be provided through a social work referral.

Day care

Day care covers a range of facilities providing for people with the mildest cognitive impairment through to severe dementia. Old people's clubs provide the lowest level of support. These are usually run by Social Services or the voluntary sector, and can provide social-isation and meals for people in the earliest stages of dementia, Day centres, usually run by Social Services, provide care for people with mild to moderate dementia, and often include transport arrangements. For patients with more severe dementia, those going through the process of diagnosis, and for people with behavioural problems, day hospi-tals provide care in a medical/nursing model. These are usually run by NHS Trusts under the supervision of either a geriatrician, an old-age psychiatrist, or occasionally run jointly.

Encouraging patients to accept day care early in the illness provides respite

for the carer, may maintain the patient in the community for longer, and can also make the transition to respite and/or residential care easier as the disease progresses.

Respite care

Respite care can be provided by either Health or Social Services. The patient is cared for in a residential care home, a nursing home or a hospital ward for periods of 1 to 6 weeks to provide the carer with a break. Social Services departments and NHS trusts usually have agreed guidelines on access to respite care and, in general, hospital-based respite care is usually reserved for patients with significant medical or behavioural problems. In some areas home-based respite care is available, allowing the carer to take a break away from home.

Long-term care

Long-term institutional care is needed when patient's can no longer be cared for in their own home, either because they live alone, or their carers are unable to cope. Health authorities, Social Services and the private sector can all provide residential care, although access to NHS continuing care is usually subject to strict guidelines based on medical need. Entry into institutional care is often a difficult and traumatic time for many patients and their carers, and support is needed to help them through this process. Access to long-term care is usually made with the support and advice of Social Services.

Genetic advice

A family history of dementia increases the risk of developing cognitive impairment in family members. In some instances, there is a clear history of autosomal dominant inheritance of dementia, where the offspring of an affected individual are at 50% risk of developing the disease. In some cases this can be attributed to mutations in presenilin, APP, tau or prion genes. For most families, however, the genetic factors increasing their risk of dementia are unknown. Many patients, their spouses and their children request advice on the genetics of dementia and it is important to provide accurate advice and formal counselling where it is needed.

It is impossible within the confines of this short book to provide detailed guidance on genetic counselling in dementia. Our general advice is to take a detailed family history to fully establish the nature of the risk to the individual. If a clear pattern of inheritance appears, particularly of young-onset disease then referral to a genetic clinic is recommended. For a more detailed discussion of genetic counselling in dementia, see Sadovnick and Lovestone (1996).

Behavioural problems

Behavioural disturbance, including aggression and agitation, is common in dementia, occurring in up to 80% of patients (Eastley et al, 1997; Jost et al, 1996; Reisberg et al, 1987; Allen and Burns, 1995). As well as being distressing to the patient, it is a significant predictor of burden in the carer, and of the need for institutionalisation (Donaldson et al, 1997).

The successful treatment of behavioural disturbance is dependent upon effecive and thorough assessment. This assessment should begin with the establishment of a definitive diagnosis, as described in the previous section, through review of all previous records to any further investigations that are needed.

Once a diagnosis is established, a full assessment of the behavioural problem should be carried out, although in some cases the diagnostic and behavioural assessments will inevitably need to occur in parallel. This part of the assessment should focus on how the behavioural problems are affecting the clinical, social and functional well-being of the patient, and what burdens are being placed on the caregiver.

An 'ABC' approach to assessing behavioural problems can be very useful in determining the frequency, association and outcomes of the problems:

A – Antecedents – What is precipitating the behaviour?
B – Behaviour – A description of exactly what the patient does.
C – Consequences – What effect does the behaviour have on the patient's, their environment and those around them.

Combining this ABC approach with a diary can provide dramatic insights into the patterns, associations and effects of the behaviour. **Figure 11** is a simple chart used by the CANDID (Counselling ANd Diagnosis in Dementia) Service (Harvey et al, 1998a) at the National Hospital to assess behavioural problems.

The primary aim of the assessment is to identify the most likely underlying cause of the behavioural problem to form the basis of an intervention. As the causes of behavioural problems in dementia are very broad, we have summarised the major causes:

- **Primary**
  - A symptom of the dementia
- **Secondary**
  - Depression
  - Anxiety
  - Psychotic illness
  - Caregiver stress/burden
- **Physical illness**
  - Infection
  - Pain
  - Sensory impairment
- **Iatrogenic (caused by the physician)**
  - Drug side-effect
  - Failure to treat a medical, surgical or psychiatric problem
- **Circumstantial**
  - Marital/relationship/disharmony
  - Frustration/boredom
  - Impaired communication
  - Elder abuse (physical or psychological)

Having established a definitive diagnosis and assessed the behavioural problems in detail, a cause and management strategy may become immediately obvious. In many cases, lack of support for the carer is a major contributing factor and, with increased support, such as with day care or respite care, the carer may find it easier to cope with the presenting problems. For other patients, an

Figure 11
Chart used by the CANDID Service to assess behavioural problems.

CANDID Behavioural Monitoring Chart

Please record **every** episode of problem behaviour. Give as much detail as possible for each episode. Note what else was going on around the patient at the time, and whether any medication was given. Record how the situation was resolved. The chart needs to be filled in for a period of not less than 14 days.

Name of client:.. Location/Contact Number:..

Date	Time	Location and who was present?	Problem behaviour	Events prior to behaviour	How was behaviour controlled?	Medication given	Notes and comments

Range of interventions

Behavioural intervention (patient or carer)	The use of behavioural or cognitive/behavioural strategy directed at either the patient, the carer or both can be helpful in managing milder behavioural problems, particularly when these are causing the carer significant stress.
Occupational activities	Engaging the patient in activities through either day care or a support/care worker can reduce boredom, and may be able to distract the patient and reduce behavioural problems.
Environmental modifications	Examples of where this type of intervention can be helpful is with patients who tend to wander; a mirror on the door will often make a wandering patient turn back, while the use of 'muddle-locks' or other security devices can prevent the patient leaving the home or getting into danger. Other environmental modifications include disconnecting gas supplies and providing pre-prepared food where gas is being left unlit. Involving an Occupational Therapist, and some imagination can often provide effective environmental solutions to common behavioural problems.
Validation therapy	The basic philosophy of validation therapy is to listen to what the patients are saying, and to validate them and what they are saying as being meaningful. Validation therapy may be helpful in patients with more severe dementia, particularly where there are also communication difficulties. Validation therapy requires training, and courses are fairly widely available.
Reminiscence therapy	Reminiscence therapy uses objects, sounds, music and discussion to provoke distant memory. The experience can be positive for patients and staff and may, at least temporarily, diminish behavioural problems.
Other	Techniques such as sensory stimulation using Snoezolem Rooms, reality orientation and other group therapies may all have a role in the management of behavioural problems.

immediate cause may not be obvious, and some general intervention will be needed.

The general principle of intervention should be to try non-pharmacological strategies first. In some situations this will not be possible. However, drug treatment should only be used following a comprehensive assessment. Simply following this process will often identify support strategies and other simple measures that can ensure the success of pharmacological treatments.

Non-pharmacological strategies

Non-pharmacological strategies cover a wide range of possibilities, although the choice will be dependent on availability and experience of staff. The broad categories that describe some of the range of interventions are listed in the box on page 86.

Pharmacological strategies

Pharmacological strategies can be divided into treating depression and treating other behavioural problems. For patients with depression, treatment is vitally important and there should be a low threshold for a trial of treatment.

Antidepressants

Antidepressants should be the first line of treatment for any patient with dementia who has signs of clinical depression. Assessing the patient's mood is an important part of the initial assessment, ideally using a formal depression rating scale, such as the BASDEC (Asdshead et al, 1992) or Cornell Scale for Depression in Dementia (Alexopoulous et al, 1988). The selective serotonin re-uptake inhibitors (SSRIs) are probably the safest drug to use as a first-line treatment. Tricyclic and related compounds should be avoided because of the potential for their anticholinergic side-effects to worsen the cognitive impairment. Starting doses should be half the usual dose, increased to a standard dose after 1 week. Patients should be given at least a 6-week trial to evaluate efficacy. Examples of suitable drugs would be:

- Paroxetine 10 mg increased to 20 mg after 1 week
- Fluoxetine 5–10 mg increased to 10–20 mg after 1 week
- Sertraline 50 mg increased to 100 mg after 1 week.

For other behavioural problems, however, professionals and carers often view the use of drugs as the simple way to fix the problem. Unfortunately, this is rarely the case and considerable caution is needed if the medication is not going to cause more problems than it solves.

The important criteria for deciding whether or not to use medication are that the problems you are attempting to treat are:

• Serious enough for drugs to be appropriate
• There are psychotic symptoms present
• The patient is experiencing significant distress
• There is a danger to the patient or others.

In any of these situations, careful consideration should be given to whether treatment can be given voluntarily without infringing the patient's rights, or whether the provisions of the Mental Health Act should be used to protect the rights of the patient and the legal position of the doctor.

Minor tranquillisers and related drugs

This group includes the benzodiazepines, carbamazepine, sodium valproate and beta-blockers. None of these drugs has been evaluated extensively for their effectiveness in managing behavioural problems in dementia and therefore caution is needed in their use. The most troublesome side-effects are usually excessive sedation, worsened confusion, ataxia, falls and occasionally a paradoxical increase in agitation and disinhibition. The starting dose should be as low as possible, certainly well below the normal starting dose, with a very gradual increase in the dose and careful monitoring of effect. The aim of treatment is firstly to ensure that the drug is having the desired effect, that any side-effects are acceptable, and that the minimum dose required to achieve the effect is being used. Treatment should also be for the shortest period possible, with the dose reduction and discontinuation at the earliest opportunity.

Neuroleptics

The conventional neuroleptics or major tranquillisers should be a last resort in the management of problem behaviour. There are very little data to confirm their efficacy, and growing evidence that they may be positively harmful to patients with dementia (McShane et al, 1997; Ballard et al, 1998), particularly those with DLB where fatal reactions to neuroleptics may occur (McKeith et al, 1992; Ballard et al, 1998). Neuroleptics are probably most effective where there are psychotic symptoms, although paradoxically these are the patients most likely to have DLB, and in whom the greatest caution is needed.

Neuroleptics with pronounced anticholinergic properties, such as thioridazine (Kirchner et al, 1998) and chlorpromazine, should particularly be avoided. High potency neuroleptics, such as haloperidol, used in very low doses (0.25 mg) has been the drug of choice, although careful monitoring for extrapyramidal side-effects is necessary. There is increasing evidence that the atypical antipsychotics, such as risperidone, olanzepine and clozapine, may be better than classical neuroleptics.

Clozapine requires careful consideration before it is used, as intensive blood monitoring is needed because of the risk of agranulocytosis.

For risperidone there is now good clinical trial evidence that treatment can result in significantly improved symptoms of psychosis and aggressive behaviour, an effect which is not linked to sedation or extrapyramidal side effects (Katz et al, 1999).

As with the minor tranquillisers, the rule should be to start at the lowest possible dose, increase very slowly, and to monitor for efficacy and side-effects ('start low and go slow'). Treatment should be short-term and should always be provided under the supervision of a specialist.

Management of specific dementias

Alzheimer's disease

Alzheimer's disease (AD) is the first degenerative dementia to have specific symptomatic drug therapy developed (Kelly et al, 1997). Treatment is based upon the neurochemical finding of reduced activity of the cholinergic marker enzyme, choline acetyltransferase, in the cerebral cortex of patients with AD. This first generation of licensed drugs is based on the use of cholinesterase inhibitors, compounds that inhibit the enzyme responsible for breaking down acetylcholine. The two most widely licensed and prescribed drugs in this class are donepezil (Rogers et al, 1998) (Aricept) and rivastigmine (Corey Bloom et al, 1998) (Exelon). The efficacy of these drugs has been assessed primarily using the Alzheimer's Disease Assessment Scale (ADAS-Cog), which assesses cognitive function and the Clinician Interview Based Impression of Change (CIBIC), which takes a global view of the patient. In large clinical trials, both drugs demonstrate modest symptomatic benefits on the ADAS-Cog and CIBIC, equivalent to a delay in symptomatic cognitive decline, together with a temporary stabilisation of the patient's clinical and functional state. It is currently unknown whether treatment has a long-term effect on delaying biological disease progression, and effects on quality of life for the sufferer and carer, and cost-effectiveness of treatment are yet to be evaluated systematically.

The lack of evidence for the effectiveness of treatment has limited the availability of treatment to patients in many countries, However, both clinical experience and responder analysis of clinical trial data suggest that, while many patients show only a limited response, up to 15–20% show much more dramatic improvements. The cautious welcome for these treatments has resulted in the development of clinical guidelines to ensure that only those patients who are benefiting receive treatment in the long term. The pharmaceutical cost of using donepezil is up to £1000 per patient per year, while the cost of rivastigmine is £650 per year.

The most influential guidelines in the UK were developed by the Department of Health's Standing Medical Advisory Committee (SMAC), these clearly state that '*it is important for clinicians not only to assess the benefits to individual patients, but also to be sensitive to the needs of the population as a whole. Resources should not be diverted to treatments whose clinical benefit and cost-effectiveness is not yet proven. A principal objective should be the avoidance of wasteful prescribing, with medicines targeted on those patients who will benefit most*'.

An array of guidelines has been published in the UK (Harvey et al, 1998), and it is possible to summarise these into pragmatic recommendations that can help clinicians wishing to assess and treat patients with AD, covering the area of: (i) patient selection and suitability; (ii) treatment initiation and monitoring; and (iii) treatment discontinuation.

Patient selection and suitability

Expert diagnosis of the patient with dementia is a prerequisite within most guidelines, and specialist referral to either an old-age psychiatrist, geriatrician or neurologist should be the initial stage when considering treatment. As a general guide, suitable patients will have mild–moderate cognitive impairment (MMSE 10–26/30), be living at home and still relatively independent, and have a reliable caregiver to supervise medication. Patients with more severe cognitive impairment, significant other medical problems, those resident in nursing homes, and patients without carers are unlikely to be suitable.

Specialist assessment will usually focus on evaluating the patient's suitability for treatment. Previous investigations will need to be reviewed, and further investigations, particularly neuroimaging and neuropsychology may be performed.

In general, suitability criteria include:

- Confirmed clinical diagnosis of probable Alzheimer's disease made using recognised criteria (DSM-IV) with a disease duration of at least 6 months
- Mild–moderate severity (MMSE score 10–26, CDR ≤2)
- Hachinski Ischaemia Score (Rosen et al, 1980) ≤ 4, to exclude significant vascular disease
- Patient able to give informed agreement to receive treatment

- Reliable caregiver available to ensure compliance
- Patient and caregiver made aware and agree to the protocol under which they will receive treatment, and that treatment will be discontinued if there is no response after 3 months
- Completion of a full clinical dementia assessment, to include neuroimaging, neuropsychology and relevant laboratory investigations, adequate to confirm the diagnosis of AD and exclude other dementias or causes for the cognitive impairment
- Absence of medical contraindications to treatment as defined in the drug information sheet.

Treatment initiation and monitoring

- Patients commence on 5 mg donepezil per day or 1.5 mg rivastigmine twice daily
- Rivastigmine dose should be increased, if tolerated, after a minimum of 2 weeks' treatment to 3 mg twice daily. Subsequent increases to 4.5 mg and then 6 mg twice daily should be based on good tolerability and may be considered after 2 weeks' treatment at each dose level.

Simple guidelines for monitoring therapy in Alzheimer's disease

Review at 6 weeks	Review at 3 months, 6 months (and then subsequently every 6–12 months)
MMSE Review of safety and tolerability (side-effects). Common side-effects with the cholinesterase inhibitors, particularly early in treatment, relate to the gastrointestinal system and include appetite loss, nausea, vomiting and diarrhoea. Temporary discontinuation or dose reduction will often diminish side-effects. Both donepezil and rivastigmine are new drugs and therefore any unusual or atypical side-effects should be reported to the Committee on Safety of Medicines (CSM) using the yellow card reporting system in the UK. If no safety or tolerability issues exist, increase dose to 10 mg donepezil per day or 6 mg rivastigmine twice daily.	MMSE Review of safety, tolerability and clinical efficacy. Clinical efficacy is probably best assessed using clinical opinion incorporating an evaluation of the patient and discussion with the carer and family. Neuropsychological assessment, functional and global rating scales may also be used as part of good clinical practice to document efficacy, although choice of assessment will be a local decision. Decision to continue or discontinue treatment

Treatment discontinuation

Treatment should be discontinued when the potential benefit of treatment (a 3–6 month delay/remission of symptoms) is no longer clinically significant in terms of the overall disease severity/stage. This will ultimately be a subjective decision made by the clinician following discussion with the patient and caregiver.

If there is doubt about the ongoing effectiveness of the drug it should be discontinued for 4–6 weeks and the usual efficacy assessments performed, including the MMSE. If there is no apparent decline then the drug should not be restarted. If there is evidence of more rapid decline following discontinuation this suggests that the drug is still effective and that it should be restarted. A trial of drug withdrawal should be considered at least every 12 months.

Poor tolerability or safety issues, poor compliance, withdrawal of consent or entry into nursing/residential care would also be indications for discontinuation.

Vascular dementia

Although a number of drug treatments are currently being assessed in clinical trials, there are so far no licensed treatments for VaD with proven efficacy. The specific treatment of VaD is therefore based on management of the underlying vascular disease and control of risk factors.

All patients with clinical VaD should undergo a through medical assessment searching for treatable vascular disease and controllable risk factors. This will include a cardiological review with a minimum of an EEG, and in many cases an echocardiogram. Doppler ultrasound or MRA should be used to exclude surgically treatable cartoid stenosis. Low-dose aspirin (150 mg daily) should be used in all patients where there is no contraindication and additional antiplatelet drugs, such as dipyridamole, if there is evidence of ongoing vascular events. Patients with multiple embolic infarcts, particularly if these have a cardiac origin, should be considered, under specialist review, for full warfarin anticoagulation. Hypertension should be adequately controlled, although considerable care is needed not to make the patient hypotensive, which may dangerously reduce blood flow to areas of the brain with critically impaired blood supply ('misery perfusion'). Blood cholesterol and triglycerides should be assessed and, if levels are significantly raised, treated using diet, drugs or both. Similarly, if the patient is diabetic, ensuring that the diabetes is well controlled is likely to be important. If the patient is a smoker, they should be encouraged to cut down or stop.

Dementia with Lewy bodies

There is some evidence that patients with DLB may respond preferentially to treatment with cholinesterase inhibitors (Levy et al, 1994; Perry et al, 1994), however, clinical trials in DLB are still ongoing to confirm this finding.

The specific management of patients with DLB mainly concerns two areas, the extrapyramidal symptoms, and the avoidance of neuroleptic drugs. If the patient with DLB has significant Parkinsonian symptoms then a trial of L-DOPA should be considered but can worsen cognition and hallucinations. Finally, as discussed in the preceding section on neuroleptic drugs, these are particularly harmful for patients with DLB. It is good practice when making a diagnosis of DLB to ensure that all other medical professionals involved, including the GP, are clear about the diagnosis and the significant risk of harm associated with the use of neuroleptics in these patients.

References

Adshead F, Day Cody D, Pitt BMN (1992) BASDEC: a novel screening instrument for depression in elderly medical patients. Available from Professor B Bitt, Memory Clinic, The Hammersmith Hospital, Ducane Road, London W12. *BMJ* **305:** 397.

Alexopoulous GS, Abrams RC, Young RC, Shamoian CA (1988) Cornell scale for depression in dementia. *Biol Psychiatry* **23:** 271–84.

Allen NHP, Burns A (1995) The non-cognitive features of dementia. *Rev Clin Gerontology* **5:** 57–75.

American Psychiatric Association (1994) *Diagnostic and Statistical Manual of Mental Disorders (4th edn) (DSM-IV).* (Washington DC: APA).

Antuono P, Doody R, Gilman E et al (1997) Diagnostic criteria for dementia in clinical trials – Position paper from the International Working Group on Harmonization of Dementia Drug Guidelines. *Alzheimer's Disease & Associated Disorders* **11(Suppl. 3):** 22–5.

Ballard C, Grace J, McKeith I, Holmes C (1998) Neuroleptic sensitivity in dementia with Lewy bodies and Alzheimer's disease. *Lancet* **351:** 1032–3.

Chiu E (1994) Huntington's Disease. In: Burns A, Levy R eds. *Dementia* (London: Chapman & Hall) 753–62.

Collinge J (1997) Human prion diseases and bovine spongiform encephalopathy (BSE). *Hum Mol Genet* **6:** 1699–705.

Copeland JR, Davidson IA, Dewey ME, Gilmore C (1992) Alzheimer's disease, other dementias, depression and pseudodementia: Prevalence, incidence and three-year outcome in Liverpool. *Brit J Psychiatry* **161:** 230–9.

Corey Bloom J, Anand R, Veach J et al (1998) A randomized trial evaluating the efficacy and safety of ENA 713 (rivastigmine tartrate), a new acetylcholinesterase inhibitor, in patients with mild to moderately severe Alzheimer's disease. *Int J Geriatric Psychopharmacol* **1:** 55–65.

Donaldson C, Tarrier N, Burns A (1997) The impact of the symptoms of dementia on caregivers. *Br J Psychiatry* **170:** 62–8.

Eastley R, Wilcock GK (1997) Prevalence and correlates of aggressive behaviours occurring in patients with Alzheimer's disease. *Int J Geriatric Psychiatry* **12:** 484–7.

Edwards G (1982) *The Treatment of Drinking Problems* (London: Grant McIntyre).

Folstein M, Folstein S, McHughs P (1975) The 'Mini Mental State': a practical method for grading the cognitive state of patients for the clinician. *J Psychiatric Res* **12:** 189–98.

Fox NC, Hartikainen P, Rossor MN (1995) Alzheimer's disease and structural imaging: CT and MRI. In: Dawbarn D, Allen SJ eds. *Neurobiology of Alzheimer's Disease* (Oxford: BIOS Scientific Publishers) 269–88.

Gearing M, Mirra SS, Hedreen JC et al (1995) The Consortium to Establish a Registry for Alzheimer's Disease (CERAD). Part X. Neuropathology confirmation of the clinical diagnosis of Alzheimer's disease. *Neurology* **45:** 461–6.

Goldman MS (1990) Experience-dependent neuropsychological recovery and the treatment of chronic alcoholism. *Neuropsychol Rev* **1:** 75–101.

Grant I (1987) Alcohol and the brain: neuropsychological correlates. *J Consulting Clin Psychol* **55**: 310–24.

Green AE, Harvey RJ, Thompson EJ, Rossor MN (1997) Increased S100 beta in the cerebrospinal fluid of patients with fronto-temporal dementia. *Neurosci Lett* **235:** 5–8.

Gurling HM, Murray RM, Ron MA (1986) Increased brain radiodensity in alcoholism: a co-twin control study. *Arch Gen Psychiatry* **43:** 764–7.

Gustafson L (1987) Frontal lobe degeneration of non-Alzheimer type II. Clinical picture and differential diagnosis. *Arch Gerontology & Geriatrics* **6:** 209–23.

Harvey RJ (1996) Review: Delusions in dementia. *Age Ageing* **25:** 405–8.

Harvey RJ (1998) A Review and Commentary on a Sample of 15 Guidelines for the Drug Treatment of Alzheimer's Disease. *Int Geriatric Psychiatry* In Press.

Harvey RJ, Roques P, Fox NC, Rossor MN (1998a) CANDID: Counselling ANd Diagnosis In Dementia. A new national service supporting the care of younger patients with dementia. *Int J Geriatric Psychiatry* **13:** 381–8.

Harvey RJ, Rossor MN, Skelton-Robinson M, Garralda ME (1998b) Young Onset Dementia: Epidemiology, clinical symptoms, family burden, support and outcome. http://dementia.ion.ucl.ac.uk/, London: Dementia Research Group.

Hill AF, Butterworth R, Joiner S et al (1999) Tonsil biopsy in the investigation of new variant CJD and other human prion diseases. *Lancet* **353:** 183–9.

Hsich G, Kenney K, Gibbs CJ et al (1996) The 14-3-3 brain protein in cerebropsinal fluid as a marker for transmissible spongiform encephalopathies. *New Engl L Med* **335:** 924–30.

Jack CR Jr (1998) Anatomic neuroimaging in dementia. In: Growden JH, Rossor MN eds. *The Dementias* (Boston: Butterworth-Heinemann) 189–218.

Jones AL, Wood JD, Harper PS (1997) Huntington disease: advances in molecular and cell biology. *J Inherited Metabolic Disease* **20:** 125–38.

Jost BC, Grossberg GT (1996) The evolution of psychiatric symptoms in Alzheimer's disease: a natural history study. *J Am Geriatrics Soc* **44**: 1078–81.

Katz IR, Jeste DV, Mintzer JE et al (1999) Comparison of risperidone and placebo for psychosis and behavioral disturbances associated with dementia: a randomized, double-blind trial. *J Clin Psych* **60**: 107–15.

Kelly CA, Harvey RJ, Cayton H (1997) Treatment for Alzheimer's disease raises clinical and ethical issues. *BMJ* **314:** 693–4.

Kennedy AM (1998) Functional neuroimaging in dementia. In: Growden JH, Rossor MN eds. *The Dementias*. (Boston: Butterworth-Heinemann) 219–55.

Kirchner V, Kelly CA, Harvey RJ (1998) A systematic review of the evidence for the safety and efficacy of thioridazine in dementia (Cochrane Review). In: Anon. *The Cochrane Library Issue 4* (Oxford: Update Software).

Kokmen E, Beard CM, Offord KP, Kurland LT (1989) Prevalence of medically diagnosed dementia in a defined United States population: Rochester, Minnesota, January 1 1975. *Neurology* **39:** 773–6.

Levy R, Eagger S, Griffiths M et al (1994) Lewy bodies and response to tacrine in Alzheimer's disease. *Lancet* **343:** 176.

Lipton SA (1997) Neuropathogenesis of acquired immunodeficiency syndrome dementia. *Curr Opin Neurol* **10:** 247–53.

Lishman WA (1997) *Organic Psychiatry: The Psychological Consequences of Cerebral Disorder* (Oxford: Blackwell Science).

McKeith I, Fairbairn A, Perry R et al (1992) Neuroleptic sensitivity with senile dementia of Lewy body type. *BMJ* **305:** 673–8.

McKeith IG, Fairbairn AF, Perry RH, Thompson P (1994) The clinical diagnosis and misdiagnosis of senile dementia of Lewy body type (SDLT). *Br J Psychiatry* **165:** 324–32.

McKeith IG, Galasko D, Kosaka K et al (1996) Consensus guidelines for the clinical and pathologic diagnosis of dementia with Lewy bodies (DLB): REport of the consortium on DLB international workshop. *Neurology* **47:** 1113–24.

McShane R, Keene J, Gedling K et al (1997) Do neuroleptic drugs hasten cognitive decline in dementia? Prospective study with necropsy follow up. *BMJ* **314:** 266–70.

Neary D, Snowden JS, Mann DM (1993) The clinical pathological correlates of lobar atrophy. *Dementia* **4:** 154–9.

Nelson HE (1991) *The National Adult Reading Test (NART) manual* 2nd edn. (Windsor: NFER-Nelson).

Perry EK, Haroutunian V, Davis KL et al (1994) Neocortical cholinergic activities differentiate Lewy body dementia from classical Alzheimer's disease. *Neuroreport* **5:** 747–9.

Pohl MI (1987) Neurocognitive impairment in alcoholics: review and comparison with cognitive impairment due to AIDS. *Adv Alcohol Subst Abuse* **7:** 107–16.

Reisberg B, Borenstein J, Salob SP et al (1987) Behavioral symptoms in Alzheimer's disease: phenomenology and treatment. *J Clin Psychiatry* **48 (Suppl.):** 9–15.

Rocca WA, Bonaiuto S, Lippi A et al (19991a) Prevalence of clinically diagnosed Alzheimer's disease and other dementing disorders. A door to door survey in Appignano, Macerata Province Italy. *Neurology* **40:** 626–31.

Rocca WA, Hofman A, Brayne C et al (1991b) The prevalence of vascular dementia in Europe – facts and fragments from 1980–1990 studies. *Annals Neurology* **30:** 817–24.

Rogers SL, Farlow MR, Mohs R et al (1998) A 24-week, double-blind, placebo-controlled trial of donepezil in patients with Alzheimer's disease. *Neurology* **50:** 136–45.

Roman GC, Tatemichi TK, Erkinjuntti T et al (1993) Vascular dementia: diagnostic criteria for research studies. Report of the NINDS-AIREN International Workshop. *Neurology* **43:** 250–60.

Rosen WG, Terry RD, Fuld PA et al (1980) Pathological verification of ischemic score in differentiation of dementias. *Annals Neurology* **7:** 486–8.

Rossor MN (1993) Alzheimer's disease. *BMJ* **307:** 779–82.

Rossor MN (1999) The dementias. In: Bradley WG, Daroff R, Fenichel G, Marsden CD eds. *Neurology in Clinical Practice.* (New York: Butterworth-Heinemann). In press.

Roth M, Tym E, Mountjoy CQ et al (1986) CAMDEX: a standarized instrument for the diagnosis of mental disorders in the elderly with reference to the early detection of dementia. *Br J Psychiatry* **149:** 698–709.

Sadovnick D, Lovestone S (1996) Genetic counselling. In: Gauthier S ed. *Clinical Diagnosis and Management of Alzheimer's Disease.* (London: Martin Dunitz Ltd) 343–58.

Sagar HJ (1998) Parkinsonian syndromes associated with dementia. In: Growden JH, Rossor MN eds. *The Dementias.* (Boston: Butterworth-Heinemann) 81–112.

Schneider JA, Watts RL, Gearing M et al (1997) Corticobasal degeneration: neuropathologic and clinical heterogeneity. *Neurology* **48:** 959–69.

Scolding NJ, Jayne DRW, Zajicek JP et al (1997) Cerebral vasculitis – recognition, diagnosis and management. *Quart J Med* **90:** 61–73.

Smith DM, Atkinson RM (1995) Alcoholism and dementia. Special issue: Drugs and the elderly: use and misuse of drugs, medicines, alcohol, and tobacco. *Int J Addict* **30 (suppl. 13–14):** 1843–69.

Suomalainen A (1997) Mitochondrial DNA and disease. *Annals Med* **29:** 235–46.

The Lund and Manchester Groups (1994) Clinical and neuropathological criteria for frontotemporal dementia. *J Neurology, Neurosurgery & Psychiatry* **57:** 416–18.

Tuck RR, Brew BJ, Britton AM, Loewy J (1984) Alcohol and brain damage. *Br J Addict* **79:** 251–9.

Verhey FR, Lodder J, Rozendaal N, Jolles J (1996) Comparison of seven sets of criteria used for the diagnosis of vascular dementia. *Neuroepidemiology* **15:** 166–72.

Victor M (1994) Alcoholic dementia. *Canad J Neurolog Sci* **21 (suppl 2):** 88–99.

Warrington EK (1989) *The Queen Square Screening Tests for Cognitive Impairment,* London: Available from The Secretary for Students, The National Hospital for Neurology and Neurosurgery, Queen Square, London WC1N 3BG, price £12.99.

Wechsler D (1981) *Manual for the Wechsler Adult Intelligence Scale – Revised* (New York Psychological Corp.).

World Health Organisation (1992) *The ICD-10 classification of mental and behavioural disorders: clinical descriptions and diagnostic guidelines* (10th edn) (Geneva: World Health Organisation).

Appendix – Voluntary organisations and support services

Alzheimer's Disease Society
Gordon House
10 Greencoat Place
London SW1P 1PH
Tel: 0171 306 0606
Fax: 0171 306 0808
Helpline 0845 300 0336
web: www.alzheimers.org.uk

Alzheimer's Scotland – Action of Dementia
Suite 269
Central Chambers
93 Hope Street
Glasgow G2 6LD
Tel/Fax: 0141 221 3854

CANDID (Counselling ANd Diagnosis in Dementia)
The National Hospital for Neurology and Neurosurgery
Queen Square
London WC1N 3BG
Tel: 0171 829 8772
Fax: 0171 209 0182
E-mail: candid@candid.ion.ucl.ac.uk
Web: candid.ion.ucl.ac.uk

Huntington's Disease Association
108 Battersea High Street
London SW11 3HP
Tel: 0171 223 7000
Fax: 0171 223 9489

Motor Neurone Disease Association UK
PO Box 246
Northamptonshire NN1 2PR
Tel: 01604 250505
Fax: 01604 24726

Parkinson's Disease Society
United Scientific House
215 Vauxhall Bridge Road
London SW1V 1EJ
Tel: 0171 931 8080
Fax: 0171 233 9908
Helpline: 0171 233 5373
(Monday – Friday 10am – 4pm)

Pick's Disease Support Group
C/O Dementia Research Group
The National Hospital for Neurology and Neurosurgery
Queen Square
London WC1N 3BG

PSP Association
The Old Rectory
Wappenham
Towcester
Northants NN12 8SQ
Tel: 01327 860299
Fax: 01327 860923
E-mail: 100572.30@compuserve.com

Stroke Association
CHSA House
Whitecross Street
London EC1Y 8JJ
Tel: 0171 490 7999
Fax: 0171 490 2686

CJD Support Network
Birchwood, Heath Top
Ashley Heath
Market Drayton
Shropshire
Tel: 01630 673 993
Helpline: 01630 673 973

Sarah Matheson Trust (Multiple System Atrophy)
Neurovascular Medicine Unit
(Pickering Unit)
Imperial College School of Medicine
St Mary's Hospital
Praed St, London W2 1NY
Tel: 0171 886 1520
Fax: 0171 886 1540

Glaxo Neurological Centre
Norton Street
Liverpool L3 8LR
Tel: 0151 298 2999
Fax: 0151 298 2333
Web: www.glaxocentre.merseyside.org

Index